Applied Tumor Immunology

Applied Tumor Immunology

Methods of Recognizing
Immune Phenomena
Specific to Tumors

Editors   Hilde Götz · E.S. Bücherl

Walter de Gruyter · Berlin · New York 1975

Proceedings of the First International Symposium, Berlin, November 1972

Prof. Dr. med. *E. S. Bücherl*, Free University of Berlin, University Hospital, Klinikum Berlin-Charlottenburg

Prof. Dr. med. *Hilde Götz*, Max-Planck-Institute for Experimental Medicine, Department of Immunochemistry

Library of Congress Cataloging in Publication Data

International Symposium on Applied Tumor Immunology, 1st,
   Berlin, 1972.
   Applied tumor immunology.

   Bibliography: XII, 355
   1. Tumors-Immunological aspects-Congresses. 2. Tumors-Diagnosis-Congresses.
3. Immunodiagnosis-Congresses. I. Götz, Hilde. II. Title.
[DNLM: 1. Antibodies, Neoplasm-Congresses. 2. Antigens, Neoplasm-Congresses.
3. Neoplasms-Immunology-Congresses. W3 IN916AE 1972a / QZ206 I615 1972a]
RC255.I52 1972 616.9'92'079 75-37806
ISBN 3-11-004242-8

CIP-Kurztitelaufnahme der Deutschen Bibliothek

Applied tumor immunology: methods of recognizing immune phenomena
specific to tumors; proceedings of the 1. Internat. Symposium, Berlin, Nov.
1972/ed. by Hilde Götz.
   ISBN 3-11-004242-8

NE: Götz, Hilde [Hrsg.]

Preface

Experimental as well as clinical findings have led to the knowledge that in case of carcinoma and in systemic malignant tumor diseases the organism's autologous immunological reactivity becomes decisive concerning the tumor cells' development and patients' fate. Basing on experiences of modern tumor immunology special methods for detecting tumor-specific immune phenomena and also concepts for an efficient immunotherapy of cancer have been developed. Although, the results of these efforts are not as yet satisfactory in clinical medicine, one should not fail to prove the applicability of efficient data from basic research work to clinical interests in the sense of "applied" tumor immunology.

It was the intention of the "1st International Symposion on Applied Tumor Immunology" held in Berlin on November 17th and 18th, 1972, reviewing the present status of this field, discussing advances in basic tumor immunology and promoting research work by mutual exchange of experience.

The symposion dealt with *problems of developing special methods for the detection of tumor-specific immune phenomena* including the interpretation of findings in clinical medicine.

The present volume records lectures and those papers that contributors submitted for publication.

We would like to present our gratitude to all speakers and participants for their contributions and for their open and fair discussions. The widespread interest of basic scientists as well as of clinical and laboratory specialists and practitioners will perhaps stimulate organizing a second symposion on this field of applied tumor immunology.

On this occasion we wish to express our thanks to the following organizations we are indebted to for financial support:

Außenamt der Freien Universität Berlin, D-1000 Berlin 33,
Bayer-Farbenfabriken AG, D-5090 Leverkusen,
C. H. Boehringer Sohn, D-6507 Ingelheim am Rhein,
Chemie Grünenthal GmbH, D-5190 Stolberg/Rhld.,
Deutsche Wellcome GmbH, D-3006 Großburgwedel,
Hoffman-La Roche AG, D-7889 Grenzach,
"medac", Gesellschaft für klinische Spezialpräparate mbH,
D-2000 Hamburg,

Rhein-Pharma, Arzneimittel GmbH, Niederlassung D-1000 Berlin 15, Schering AG, D-1000 Berlin 65.

We would finally like to thank the secretary of the symposion, Mrs L. Weinberger and her helpers and the interpreter group of Mrs. D. Helmrich.

Though, the contributions of the symposion in 1972 come out but now, most of the papers were brought to the recent state of knowledge.

Berlin and Göttingen, October 1975   The Organizing Committee

Prof. Dr. med. *E. S. Bücherl*
Prof. Dr. med. *Hilde Götz*

Contents

List of Contributors

1. Albrecht, R.
2. Baldi, C.
3. Bansal, S. C.
4. Bauder, E. L.
5. Bauer, H.
6. Benso, L.
7. Biarese, V.
8. Bonardi, R.
9. Brendel, W.
10. Brunet, R. M.
11. Diehl, V.
12. Dietmair, E.
13. Fischer, K.
14. Gelderblom, H.
15. Götz, H.
16. Grundmann, E.
17. Guarini, G.
18. Hermann, G.
19. Iudicello, P.
20. Jacob, R. M.
21. Kleist von, S.
22. Knight, R. A.
23. Koldovský, P.
24. Kurth, R.

25. Lampert, F.
26. Lischner, H.
27. Lovisetto, P.
28. Mach, J. P.
29. Molfese, G.
30. Nagel, E.
31. Nagel, G. A.
32. Nigro, N.
33. Pappas, A.
34. Poschmann, A.
35. Prokop, O.
36. Pusztaszeri, G.
37. Ricci, C.
38. Ring, J.
39. Robinson, E.
40. Rothe, A.
41. Scheurlen, P. G.
42. Schneider, C. C.
43. Schultze-Mosgau, H.
44. Smith, J. B.
45. Uebel, H.
46. Uhlenbruck, G.
47. Warnatz, H.
48. Weinstein, J.

List of Invited Active Participants

1. *Bansal*, S. C., M. D., Department of Surgery, Medical College of Pennsylvania, 3300 Henry Ave., Philadelphia, Penn. 19129, U.S.A.
2. *Benso*, L., Prof., Clinica Pediatrica, Università di Torino, Piazza Polonia, 94, I-10121 Torino, Italy.
3. *Brendel*, W., Prof. Dr. med. Dr. hc., Institut für Chirurgische Forschung an der Chirurgischen Klinik der Universität München, Nußbaumstraße 20, D-8000 München, Germany.
4. *Bücherl*, E. S., Prof. Dr. med., Chirurgische Universitätsklinik und -Poliklinik im Klinikum Charlottenburg der Freien Universität Berlin, Spandauer Damm 130, D-1000 Berlin 19, Germany.
5. *Diehl*, V., Priv.-Doz. Dr. med., Abteilung Hämatologie und Onkologie, Medizinische Hochschule Hannover, Karl-Wiechert-Allee 9, D-3000 Hannover-Kleefeld, Germany.
6. *Fischer*, K., Prof. Dr. med., Abteilung für Klinische Immunpathologie, Universitäts-Kinderklinik und -Poliklinik Hamburg-Eppendorf, Martinistraße 52, D-2000 Hamburg 20, Germany.
7. *Gallmeier*, W. M., Priv.-Doz. Dr. med., Innere Klinik und Poliklinik (Tumorforschung), Klinikum Essen der Ruhr-Universität Bochum, Städtische Krankenanstalten, Hufelandstraße 55, D-4300 Essen-Holsterhausen, Germany.
8. *Gelderblom*, H., Dr. med., Robert-Koch-Institut Berlin, Nordufer 20, D-1000 Berlin 65, Germany.
9. *Götz*, H., Prof. Dr. med., Abteilung Immunchemie, Max-Planck-Institut für experimentelle Medizin, Hermann-Rein-Straße 3, D-3400 Göttingen, Germany.
10. *Grundmann*, E., Prof. Dr. med., Pathologisches Institut der Universität Münster, Westring 17, D-4400 Münster, Germany.
11. *Guarini*, G., Prof., Istituto di Clinica Medica Generale e Terapia Medica, Università di Torino, Corso Polonia, 14, I-10121 Torino, Italy.
12. *Hermann*, G., Prof. Dr. Dr. med., Immunologische Abteilung, Chirurgische Universitätsklinik Köln, Robert-Koch-Straße 10, D-5000 Köln, Germany.
13. *Hilschmann*, N., Prof. Dr. med., Abteilung Immunchemie, Max-Planck-Institut für experimentelle Medizin, Hermann-Rein-Straße 3, D-3400 Göttingen, Germany.

14. *Kleist* von, S., Dr. med., Laboratoire d'Immunochimie, Institut de Recherches Scientifiques sur le Cancer, 7, Rue Guy-Mocquet, F-94800 Villejuif, France.

15. *Koldovský*, P., Prof., M. D., The Joseph Stokes, Jr., Research Institut, The Children's Hospital of Philadelphia, 34th Street and Civic Center Boulevard, Philadelphia, PA. 19104, U.S.A.

16. *Kurth*, R., Dr. med., Friedrich Miescher-Laboratorium, Max Planck-Gesellschaft, Spemannstraße 37–39, D-7400 Tübingen, Germany.

17. *Lampert*, F., Prof. Dr. med., Kinderklinik der Justus Liebig-Universität, Feulgenstraße 12, D-6300 Gießen, Germany.

18. *Lovisetto*, P., Prof., Instituto di Clinica Medica Generale e Terapia Medica, Università di Torino, Corso Polonia, 14, I-10121 Torino, Italy.

19. *Mach*, J.-P., Dr. med., Institut de Biochimie, Université de Lausanne, 21, Rue du Bugnon, CH-1011 Lausanne, Switzerland.

20. *Macher*, E., Prof. Dr. med., Hautklinik der Westfälischen Wilhelms-Universität, von-Esmarch-Straße 56, D-4400 Münster, Germany.

21. *Mayersbach* von, H., Prof. Dr. med., Institut für Anatomie, Abteilung I, Medizinische Hochschule Hannover, Karl-Wiechert-Allee 9, D-3000 Hannover-Kleefeld, Germany.

22. *Nagel*, G. A., Priv.-Doz. Dr. med., Abteilung für Onkologie, 1. Medizinische Universitätsklinik, Departement für Innere Medizin, CH-4004 Basel, Switzerland.

23. *Pappas*, A., Prof. Dr. med., Medizinische Universitätsklinik und -Poliklinik, Innere Medizin I, D-6650 Homburg, Germany.

24. *Pilch*, Y. H., Ass. Prof. M. D., Department of Surgery, School of Medicine, The Center for the Health Sciences, Los Angeles, California 90024, U.S.A.

25. *Poschmann*, A., Priv.-Doz. Dr. med., Abteilung für Klinische Immunpathologie, Universitäts-Kinderklinik Hamburg-Eppendorf, Martinistraße 52, D-2000 Hamburg 20, Germany.

26. *Prokop*, O., Prof. Dr. med., Institut für gerichtliche Medizin der Humboldt-Universität Berlin, Hannoversche Straße 6, DDR-104 Berlin, German Democratic Republic.

27. *Pusztaszeri*, G., Dr. med., Institut de Biochimie, Université de Lausanne, 21, Rue du Bugnon, CH-1011 Lausanne, Switzerland.

28. *Ricci*, C., Prof., Istituto di Clinica Medica Generale e Terapia Medica, Università di Torino, Corso Polonia, 14, I-10126 Torino, Italy.

29. *Robinson*, E., Prof., Department of Oncology, The Aba Khoushy School of Medicine, Rambam Government Hospital, Haifa, Israel.

30. *Schneider*, C. C., Dr. rer. nat., Biologisches Institut – Dr. Madaus & Co. Köln, Ostmerheimer Straße 198, D-5000 Köln-Merheim 91, Germany.

31. *Schultze-Mosgau*, H., Priv.-Doz. Dr. med., Frauenklinik des Universitäts-krankenhauses Hamburg-Eppendorf, Martinistraße 52, D-2000 Hamburg 20, Germany.
32. *Seiler*, W., Dr. med., Abteilung für Onkologie, 1. Medizinische Univer-sitätsklinik, Departement für Innere Medizin, CH-4004 Basel, Switzer-land.
33. *Smith*, J. B., M. D., University College London, Gower Street, GB-London WCI E 6BT, Great Britain.
34. *Uhlenbruck*, G., Prof. Dr. med., Abteilung für Immunbiologie, Medizi-nische Universitätsklinik Köln, Kerpener Straße 15, D-5000 Köln 41, Germany.
35. *Warnatz*, H., Prof. Dr. med., Institut und Poliklinik für klinische Immu-nologie der Universität Erlangen-Nürnberg, Krankenhausstraße 12, D-8520 Erlangen, Germany.

1 Methods for Detection of Tumor-Specific Sensitized Lymphocytes

1.1 Tumor-Specific and Cell-Mediated Immune Reactions Expressed in Pathomorphological Findings

E. Grundmann

Three separate processes can be distinguished during oncogenesis (1):

1. The initiation, i. e. the transformation of normal somatic cells into cancer cells,
2. the extension of the tumor promoted by excessive growth,
3. the escape of tumor tissue from endogenous regulations leading finally to the death of the patient.

Immunologic reactions are involved in each of them, but their respective value is unequal.

The primary process is a matter of molecular biology. Chemical carcinogens, for example, will transform DNA-bases by way of metabolic products. Diazoalkane could be mentioned as an instance: produced by hydroxylation and heterolysis of dialkylenitrosamines (2), it can methylize the guanine of the DNA double helix. The reaction of "terminal cancerogenes" (i. e. dialkane in this case) with a transfer-RNA by means of a transfer-RNA-methylase may be more important than a direct methylation of guanine (3). Oncogenic RNA-viruses are able to transform DNA by an intermediate of invert transscriptase, a RNA-dependent DNA-polymerase.

This primary process has to be mentioned first because of its considerable importance in tumor immunology. We know today that cancer cells, be they induced by chemical agents or by viruses, will be recognized as "strangers" by the tumor host, and will be treated accordingly. This may be the consequence of an antigen defect or of newly arising antigens. Neo-antigens have been found particularly in experimentally induced viral cancers.

They can be of viral nature determined by specificity of viral nucleic acids. If an organism possesses beforehand antibodies for the specific virus, the primary process can be suppressed. Experimental evidence can be obtained by viral infection, or even by injection of irradiated cells from viral tumors: the animals are specifically virus-resistent. The meaning of such immunities against certain tumor viruses and its impact on human oncogenesis, are rather vague for the time being. Principally, the primary process of cancerization appears controlled by immunologic mechanisms.

Practical evidence of a malignant tumor cannot be obtained before it has entered the second stage, the growth phase. Immunological reactions are more easily grasped in this phase, and that is why almost every approach to tumor immunology starts here. When murine or rodent tumors are grafted on isogeneic animals, excessive growth will start immediately. In allogeneic or heterogeneic animals growth will stop after a few days, and tumors disappear. Heterologous transplantation of JENSEN-sarcoma from rats to mice is an adequate example: tumors are growing until day 11 after grafting, then they turn necrotic and are rejected. Histologically, the process is accompanied by an infiltration of lymphocytes and plasma cells surrounding the transplant (Fig. 1). This inflammatory wall was known for quite some time (4) and was called "Immunitätsgewebe" by WALLBACH (5). It is found in most malignant tumors. In histodiagnostical practice we may go by the formula: Many lymphocytes indicate slow progress, fewer lymphocytes mean rapid growth of a tumor. Such a rule of thumb has, of course, to be taken with all necessary precautions.

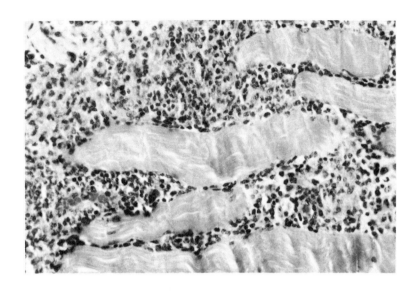

Fig. 1. Abundant lymphocytic infiltration after heterologous
transplant of JENSEN-sarcoma to the mouse. Many lymphocytes,
but only a few tumor cells preserved among muscle fibres.
Typical graft rejection. HE x 320.

Three model cases can be described:

A basalioma must be defined as malignant skin tumor on account
of its primary process. It is surrounded by a dense wall of lymphocytes with many histiocytes which are some times accumula-
ted in small knots (Fig. 2). Histologically, this "Immunitätsgewebe" presents an analogy to graft rejection in an allogeneic
transplant, for instance of a skin graft in mice (6).

In terms of morphology, female chorion carcinoma is an
example for the opposite. This tumor owes an exceptional position in oncology to the fact that it is a human transplantation
tumor, indeed. When it is left untreated, rapid local and massed
metastatic growth will lead to death in most cases. Even the
earlier chorial invasion into the placenta is completely free
from lymphocytes, and the same phenomenon is often seen in

the full grown tumor and its metastases. - The most simple explanation would be that the mother had acquired immune-tolerance against embryonal cells. As the problem does not exactly belong to my topic, it will not be considered for the moment; but it may be of interest that chorial carcinomas can spontaneously regress when lymphocytes are abounding in their immediate vicinity.

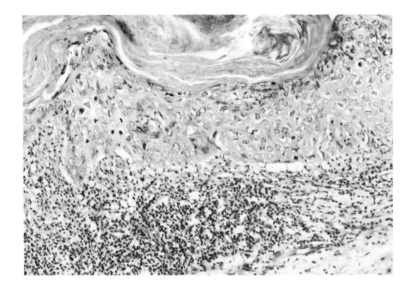

Fig. 2. Morbus BOWEN with intense lymphocytic reaction below intraepithelial carcinoma cells. HE x 130.

Lymphogranulomatosis provides a third example in pathological histology. Following LUKES and Coll. (7), Morbus HODGKIN today is staged in at least 4 histologic types: the lymphocytic predominant type, the mixed lymphocytic-histiocytic type, the lymphocytic depleted type, and nodular sclerosis (the latter might possibly be seen as a disease sui generis). We have to emphasize that in the first three types histologic features will undoubtedly

determine both clinical development and prognosis. The lymphocytic predominant type grows slowly and can remain almost sta-
tionary for years - in some cases even for decades. The mixed
type corresponds, seen under clinical and morphological aspects,
to the classical picture of M.HODGKIN whereas the lymphocytic
depleted type has the shortest mean life expectancy. Histologically the latter is called "HODGKIN sarcoma" for its likeness to the
reticulum cell sarcoma. Here again the limits of my theme prevent detailed consideration of the problems in primary malignancy of M.HODGKIN. However, it stands for certain that a case of
lymphocytic predominance can turn into lymphocytic depletion,
which actually means increased malignancy. This way an initially
slow growing neoplasm can change to rapid proliferation, whereas
the reverse, i. e. transition from lymphocytic depletion to lymphocytic predominance, has never been found.
Chemotherapy enhances the transformation toward the depleted
type. All cytostatic agents have a lymphocyte-destructive effect -
we shall go into that later.

It should be explained first whether this wall of lymphocytes observed in the neighbourhood of tumor cells (WALLBACH's "Immunitätsgewebe", 5) is in fact the cause, or merely a sequel of
tumor regression or arrested growth. For quite a while it was
maintained that these lymphocytes were expressing a reaction on
cell-destruction inside the tumor or in its immediate environment
(8). Our team with MADAUS and HOBIK (9) has refuted this opinion. An antilymphocytic serum against murine lymphocytes was
produced in rabbits and then tried on mice which had received
heterologous grafts of rats JENSEN-sarcoma. The mice were given a daily dose of 0, 2 ml antilymphocytic serum for 12 days.
From day 9 after the grafting of JENSEN-sarcoma, the heterolo-

gous tumors started to grow rapidly in the ALS-treated mice.
Controls which were given either saline or a similar dose of
normal rabbit serum, showed complete tumor regression during
the same time (Fig. 3).

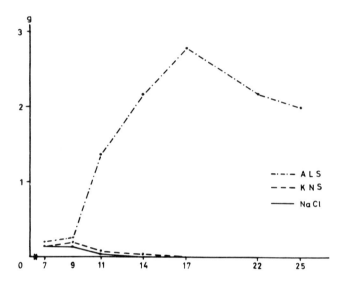

Fig. 3. Tumor weights of rat JENSEN-sarcoma after heterologous grafting on the mouse under ALS, and treatment with normal rabbit serum (KLS), and under treatment with NaCl. Animals treated with ALS attain a maximum tumor weight of 2,7 g
on day 17 (cf. GRUNDMANN, MADAUS and HOBIK, 1969).

Lymphocytes in the peripheral blood of controls remained constant, while the ALS-treated animals showed a characteristic
lymphopenia as an immediate consequence. Histologically, no
lymphocytic reaction whatever was found in the tumor surrounding tissue of the ALS-treated animals (Fig. 4). It was further interesting that mitosis counts in controls had recorded normal
mitotic rates until day 9, and rapid decrease after that, whereas
the ALS-treated animals showed a remarkable increase in mitotic rates. Here too, growth declined rapidly after day 7.

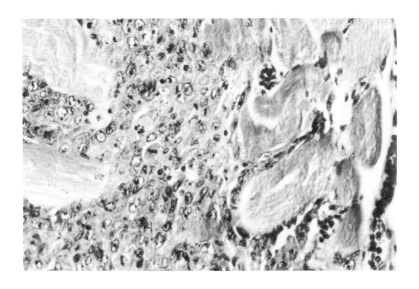

Fig. 4. Rat JENSEN-sarcoma in heterologous graft on a mouse.
Host treated with ALS. No graft rejection. HE x 320.

ALS treatment was stopped after 12 days - the mice had tumors
of some 3 g - and rapid rejection of tumors followed. In these
experiments, tumors behaved like any other heterologous graft -
and that is what they actually are.

This experience led to studies of human tumors analyzing in detail the intensity of lymphocytic reaction and its correlation to
tumor growth. Our results were as follows:
The majority of cells invading the neighbourhood of a carcinoma
are smaller and bigger lymphocytes, plasma cells and histiocytic macrophages. Squamous carcinoma of the larynx is shown as
an example (Fig. 5). In areas densely populated by lymphocytes
mitoses are very rare. Many tumor cells are destroyed, symptoms of cytolysis and pyknosis are found. In lymphocytic depleted
parts tumor cells are well preserved and frequently mitotic.
These are the growth zones of the carcinoma. It happens not

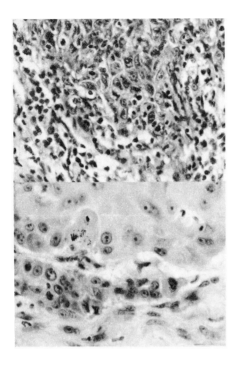

Fig. 5. Tumor cones in squamous cell carcinoma of larynx. Top: slow growing tumor zone with many plasma cellular lymphocytes and histiocytes. Bottom: fast growing tumor zone (zone of intense tumor growth) without inflammatory infiltration. HE x 200.

infrequently that lymphocytic predominance and depletion are found in close vicinity. What is the interpretation of these findings? Transplant immunology has shown that of all the lymphocytes invading an allograft, the "activated" ones make but a small proportion. This relative scarcity of "active" lymphocytes allows an immunologic defense reaction in only a few areas of the carcinoma growth front. The military metaphor is quite adequate: malignant tumor cells are the aggressors, and the defense relies on rather a limited number of soldiers. The defenders try to obviate and stop aggression in some places at least; but the aggressor with his superior force will go rapidly

forward in all parts denuded of defenders. Thus, tumor growth
appears to reflect the ever changing balance between powers of
aggression and powers of defense. The evaluation of such observations entitles us to adopt our "rule of thumb" in histological
diagnostics, too: many lymphocytes in the neighbourhood of a
tumor are a sign of adequate, few lymphocytes indicate a poor
tumor defence. FISHER and FISHER /Pittsburgh (10) have demonstrated this relation in a very elegant experimental model.
Tumors were induced in rats with methylcholanthrene, and then
grafted to isogeneic or allogeneic rats below the renal capsule.
In isogeneic transplants to LEWIS rats there was no lymphocytic
infiltration; tumors grew rapidly and unimpeded. In allogeneic
transplants to BUFFALO rats there was an intensive lymphocytic
infiltration that started five days after tumor grafting. Some of
the LEWIS rats had got the same tumors implanted subcutaneously two weeks before. Another group of LEWIS rats was prepared in the same way, but the implanted tumor was removed
immediately before the grafting into kidneys. The first group of
rats was called concomitants, the other sinecomitants. In both
of them the previous grafting with the same tumor had provoked
a sensitization. The tumor grafts into the kidneys failed to grow
and were surrounded by dense lymphocytic infiltration. But here
too, antilymphocyte serum was able to suppress this lymphocytic
infiltration.

The vital role of lymphocytes was proved in several experiments
where tumor immunity was shown to be inactively transferred by
sensitized lymphocytes. BRUNNER (11) utilized DBA/2 ascites
tumor cells; the growth rate of tumors was determined by cell
count in the ascites   or by registering the animals' lethality.
In lethally irradiated mice pretreated with isogeneic C3H- lym-

phocytes, protection against allogeneic tumor cells would depend
on lymphocyte donors being previously immunized by identical
tumor cells. In another experimental series lethally irradiated
C3H mice received once more lymphocytes sensitized against
DBA/2 tumor cells, in order to rebuild their immunity. After
that, the animals were intraperitoneally injected a mixture of
allogeneic DBA/2 tumor cells and isogeneic C3H tumor cells.
While the allogeneic tumor cells were completely destroyed,
lymphocytes being sensitized against them, the simultaneously
injected syngeneic tumor cells continued their growth unchecked.
It follows that no unspecific mechanism was contributing to the
immune reaction which had been passively transferred by lymphocytes.

In a third series BRUNNER (11) and his collaborators have pretreated these immune lymphocytes with antithcta serum with
complement. Such a destruction of thymus dependent lymphocytes was shown to eventually delete all immunologic protection.

The well established definition in transplant immunology was
thus safely ascertained for tumor immunology: The "activated"
lymphocytes are T-lymphocytes, i.e. of the thymus dependent
form.

In this context the question is raised as to which might be the
role of the thymus itself in tumor immunology. We have examined the problem in several experimental series with mice.

When fed diethylnitrosamine, mice like rats will develop liver
carcinomas. Neonatal thymectomy remains without influence,
neither on latency periods nor on tumor frequency (HOBIK,
unpubl.). Even the primary growth of tumor grafts was not
significantly influenced by neonatal thymectomy. In contrast,
the development of pulmonary adenomas induced by

7, 12-dimethylbenzanthrazene revealed an undoubted correlation. Within 32 weeks following treatment, pulmonary adenomas arose in non-thymectomized animals at a rate of 53%, in neonatally thymectomized animals at 91%. For controls, the average number of tumors (adenomas) was 0, 53% in normal, but 3, 3% in thymectomized animals. Without treatment on dimethylbenzanthracene, the rate of spontaneous and of postthymectomy adenomas was negligible.

In experimental breast carcinomas the result of thymectomy was not an increase, but a decrease of tumor incidence (12). Therefore it is not easy to find a common denomination for the role of the thymus. The general spread of T-lymphocytes in an organism is probably completed at birth. After that, a removal of the thymus as productive or formative organ, would be of no further consequence.

Nevertheless, the problem has its bearing on human pathology. PAPATESTAS and his colleagues (13) have published some remarkable results obtained at Mount Sinai Hospital/New York. They subjected to a retrospective study all cases of myasthenia gravis treated in that hospital between 1951 and 1971. The material comprised the impressive number of 1243 patients. 140 of them, i. e. 11%, had developed neoplasms after the onset of the basic disease. Of these neoplasms, 46 were malignant thymomas, 94 were tumors located in other organic sites. For the moment, the correlation of thymus tumors and myasthenia gravis will be-left aside. The massed incidence of extrathymal tumors seems to be of greater interest: 25 among them (27%) were breast carcinomas. Tumors of the respiratory system appeared at the rather small rate of 10%. 60% of the patients were women, 40% men. It may be further interesting that most of the tumors arose immediately after the onset of the basic disease. Until 19 years after this onset, the average tumor rate among these patients was considerably higher than in a control group adjusted to the persons under observation. In patients who had been thymectomized as treatment of myasthenia gravis, the rate of malignant extrathymal tumors went down to that found in normal controls within five years.

There is a possible correlation to experimental findings:
In animals with congenital or acquired immunodeficiencies, malignant tumor incidence appears markedly increased, especially that of lymphoreticular sarcomas. NEW ZEALAND mice can be mentioned here which were introduced in literature by BIELSCHOWSKY and coll. (14) as NZB or NZW mice. These animals bear a genetic deficiency and fall - at the age of 6-10 months, victims of an autoimmune disease under symptoms of dermatitis, splenomegaly and glomerulosclerosis like in lupus erythematodes - often with signs of hemolytic anemia. Lymphoreticular sarcomas were observed in these animals in 40% of cases (Fig. 6).

Another experimentally induced status of disturbed immunity appears in the graft-vs-host reaction when the graft is turning "against" its host. Dr. HOBIK of our team used the model of SIMONSEN (15): $C_{57}Bl/6$ males were mated with Balb/c females. The F_1-hybrids receive each, at the age of 10 days, an intraperitoneal injection of 3-18 x 10^6 spleen cells taken from males of the $C_{57}bl/6$ strain. These paternal spleen cells settle in the receptor's spleen and start to proliferate, inducing an immunological reaction. The animals' habitus is like that after neonatal thymectomy, and they die rather soon of this "runt-disease". When they can be kept alive for some months, the majority will

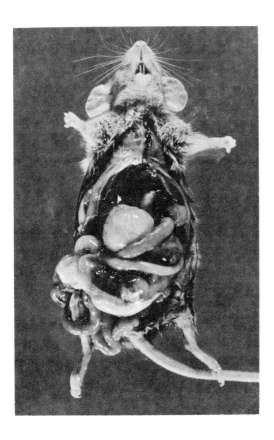

Fig. 6. NZB/NZW mouse with spontaneous abdominal malignant lymphomas (H. P. HOBIK, unpublished).

have developed lymphoreticular sarcomas - in Dr. HOBIK's
series it was 78, 3%.

In both models the viral origin of lymphoreticular sarcomas
plays an important role. We have to assume that partial disturbance of the immunologic balance between the viral antigen
and the host's reaction, will provoke progressive cell proliferation especially in the lymphoreticular tissues. KRÜGER (16)
has seen the lymphoreticular reaction as an attempted compen-
sation or pseudocompensation which, under incomplete neutra-
lizytion of antigens, results in a circulus vitosus leading to-

wards neoplasia. The immunosuppressive effect of leukemia viruses - demonstrated in our team by SEIDEL and LAUENSTEIN (17) - is apt to enhance the development.

Studies in human pathology have also realized how congenital immunodeficiencies would lead to an increase in reticuloendothelial tumors. An example is found in the LOUIS-BAR-syndrome (ataxia-teleangiectasia) where some 10% of the affected children will die of lymphoreticular sarcomas (18). In lupus erythematodes (18), in autoimmune hemolytic anemia, and even in rheumatoid arthritis, the rate of lymphoreticular sarcomas is higher than in comparable control groups. In most of these diseases histologic findings will often show hyperplasia of thymus with follicular centres and occasional thymomas (19).

Here again we have to mention the effect of cytostatic agents used in therapy which is also immunosuppressive in most of them. Long lasting immunosuppressive treatment - e.g. after renal transplantation - increases the risk of the patient developing malignant tumors. PENN (20) made an investigation of 3000 renal transplantation patients wherein he reported 37 malignant tumors within rather a short period, among them 12 reticulum cell sarcomas. More recent studies establish a safe rate of tumors at 6%. All cases were excluded where tumor cells of donors could possibly be transmitted by way of the renal graft.

The slogan of "immunologic surveillance" was very aptly coined to describe the whole concept. As far as I know, the word was introduced by THOMAS (21) and adopted and extended by several other teams (BURNET, 22). The term "immunologic surveillance" is based on the behaviour of certain carcinomas which start rather frequently in the organism of elderly people, but are checked and stopped immediately by the immunologic "police force". The latter is recruited of lymphocytes that are capable to stop and suppress completely the growth of a tumor. Thus, the actual and final manifestation of a malignant tumor would be the consequence of failing immunologic surveillance.

Any concept deduced mainly from experimental results needs revising and confirmation in human pathology. We shall have to look carefully for pointers to immunologic surveillance in humans. The facts mentioned first with regard to the balance of aggression and defence at the tumor growth front could furnish histologic evidence for this concept. Some special problems are found in close correlation. It has been observed that gastric carcinomas possess no particular wall of lymphocytes in the immediate neighbourhood, although the gastric mucosa is originally well equipped with lymphocytes. The discrepancy is easily explained by the role of gastro-intestinal lymphoreticular tissue: it is seen as potential source, or field of activity of B-lymphocytes, but not of the T-lymphocytes on which tumor immunity mostly depends. The absence of T-lymphocytes and the remarkable early metastatic tendency in gastric carcinomas would suggest causal correlation. The number of original "native" T-lymphocytes in the stomach may be so small as to allow no effective local tumor rejection at all, or merely a very limited one. This immunologic aspect would help to explain the extremely fast progress of many gastric carcinomas and the resulting high mortality. In Germany, even today, nearly half of all gastric carcinomas are in a stage of practical inoperability when surgical intervention is started; the mean survival expectancy of tumor patients after surgery is still less than two years.

Another example taken from human pathology: An investigation of LIAVAG (23) stated latend prostate carcinomas in more than 20% of all men over 50. The rate is age-dependent and goes up to 66, 7% in the age group of 90-99 years.

The term "latent carcinoma" implies that these tumors have not attained their full growth, possibly being checked by the "immunologic surveillance".

Nevertheless, the theory of immunologic surveillance goes not uncontested. Five arguments can be cited for the opposite side:

1. In animals and in humans immunologic disturbance provokes mostly lymphoreticular sarcomas. The majority of human malignant tumors are, however, carcinomas.

2. When chemical carcinogens are tested in animal experiments under simultaneous immunosuppression, tumor incidence is not increased (24).

3. ALS can also stop the "catching" of malignant tumors. This was the result of LAPPE and BLAIR (25) in their study of spontaneous mamma tumors in mice.

4. In our investigations of cancer cytogenesis we found no experimental evidence of so-called "resting" cancer cells. Even minute clones ot tumor cells arising in liver, skin or thyroid under effect of cancerogenic substances, would start growing immediately, while a lymphocytic wall was only subsequently developed (26, 27). Female carcinoma in situ at the portio uteri shows, as a rule, no infiltration of lymphocytes at all, or only a very restricted one. The lymphocytic infiltration will never set in before a deep invasive progress of malignant growth.

5. Immunologic reactions are not always and altogether detrimental to tumor growth. Antibodies may neutralize immuno-

competent lymphocytes, thereby favorizing the progress of tumor growth. This is called the "enhancement phenomenon" which has acquired increasing importance in tumor immunology.

Let me summarize:

Experimental and human pathology have secured pints in favor of the concept of "immunologic surveillance". T-lymphocytes are in fact capable to dissolve or destroy tumor cells in vivo. Absence of lymphocytes enhances and accelerates tumor growth. The progress of a tumor appears as an expression of the local defeat of T-lymphocytes. Histologic evidence could support this. In most cases the immunosystem is not able to assert itself against the proliferative power of malignant cells. In tumor patients the balance between biological growth potential of tumor cells and immunologic surveillance is declined in favor of malignancy.

References

1. GRUNDMANN, E. (1972), Verh. Deut. Ges. Inn. Med. 78, 34.

2. SCHMÄHL, D. (1970), Entstehung, Wachstum und Chemotherapie maligner Tumoren, Editio Cantor KG, Aulendorf/Württ.

3. MAGEE, P.N. (1974), Recent Results Cancer Res. 44, 2.

4. RIBBERT, H. (1916), Deut. Med. Wochenschr. 10, 278.

5. WALLBACH, G. (1929), Z. Krebsforsch. 29, 577.

6. GRUNDMANN, E. (1970), Verh. Deut. Ges. Pathol. 54, 65.

7. LUKES, R.J., CRAVER, L.F., HALL, T.C., RAPPAPORT, H. & RUBIN, P. (1966), CANCER Res. 26, 1311.

8. HACKMANN, Ch. (1950), Z. Krebsforsch. 57, 164.

9. GRUNDMANN, E., MADAUS, W.P. & HOBIK, H.P. (1969), Beitr. Pathol. Anat. 140, 89.

10. FISHER, E.R. & FISHER, B. (1972), Arch. Pathol. 94, 137.

11. BRUNNER, K.T. (1972), Schweiz. Med. Wochenschr. 102, 1144.

12. ALLISON, A. C. & TAYLOR, R. B. (1967), Cancer Res. 27, 703.

13. PAPATESTAS, A. E., OSSERMANN, K. E. & KARK, A. E. (1972), Brit. J. Cancer 25, 635.

14. BIELSCHOWSKY, M., HELYER, B. J. & HOWIE, J. B. (1959), Proc. Univ. Otago Med. School 37, 9.

15. SIMONSEN, M.   (1962), Progr. Allergy 6, 349

16. KRÜGER, G. (1971), Verh. Deut. Ges. Pathol. 55, 200.

17. SEIDEL, H. J. & LAUENSTEIN, K. (1969), Z. Krebsforsch. 72, 219.

18. ALEXANDER, J. W. & GOOD, R. A. (1970), Immunology of Surgeons. Saunders, Philadelphia.

19. MILLER, J. F. A. P., GRANT, G. A. & ROE, F. J. C. (1963), Nature (London) 199, 920.

20. PENN, I. (1970), Recent Results Cancer Res. 35, 1.

21. THOMAS, L. (1959), Cellular and Humoral Aspects of the Hypersensitive State (ed. Lawrence, H. S.), p. 529, Hoeber, New York, U.S.A.

22. BURNET, F. M. (1970), Immunological Surveillance, Pergamon Press, Oxford.

23. LIAVAG, J., HARBITZ, T. B. & HAUGEN, O. A. (1972), Recent Results Cancer Res. 39, 131.

24. SCHMÄHL, D., WAGNER, R. & SCHERF, H. R. (1971), Arzneim.-Forsch. (Drug Res.) 21, 403.

25. LAPPÉ, M. A. & BLAIR, P. B. (1970), Proc. Amer. Assoc. Cancer Res. 11, 47.

26. GRUNDMANN, E. & SIEBURG, H. (1962), Beitr. Pathol. Anat. 126, 57.

27. GRUNDMANN, E. & SEIDEL, H. J. (1965), Beitr. Pathol. Anat. 132, 188.

1.2 Problems in Identifying Tumor-Specific Sensitized Lymphocytes

S. C. Bansal

Introduction

The lymphoid system which is responsible for defending the host from external and internal hostile assaults, such as from mycobacteria, viruses, bacteria, allografts and aberrant neoplastic transformed cells (immunological surveillance), can respond in a non-specific manner as well as specifically to any assault on the host. At least two functionally distinct specific responses to an antigenic stimulus are recognized (Table 1).

Table 1: Specific responses of lymphoid system

a) Cell-Mediated Immune Response (i. e., cell-mediated possibly thymus-dependent cells)

1) Delayed hypersensitivity

2) Homograft rejection

b) Humoral Immune Response (by formation of immunoglobulin of various classes, e.g., IgM, IgG, IgA, etc., which may have the following biological functions)

1) Complement-dependent cytotoxic response

2) Non-complement-dependent blocking of cell-mediated immunity --blocking serum factors(1-3)

3) Non-complement-dependent abrogation of blocking serum factors--unblocking serum factors (1-4)

4) Cytophilic, arming of non-sensitized lymphocytes (5)

5) Antibody induced cell-mediated immunity (in vitro) by unsensitized lymphocytes (13).

The general question of host defense in animals and human cancer is presently a subject of intense investigation. During the
last decade, a growing amount of information from various laboratories has indicated the critical role of the systemic immune
response in a tumor-bearing host (6-10). The information available from these investigations indicates that both experimental
tumors in animals and spontaneous tumors in humans exhibit
weak antigenic response in the host of origin. Efforts have been
made do define tumor-specific antigens and to obtain in vivo and
in vitro evidence that the tumor-bearing host responds to these
tumor-specific antigens by both cellular and humoral responses.
Many recent reviews covering these aspects lead to the conclusion that host immune factors in a tumor-bearing host are, in
fact, involved in inhibition or progression of its tumor (reviews
6-10, 12). Our knowledge of such immune responses has increased enormously during the last few years with the introduction of methods for analyzing them in vitro (11).

The tumor-bearing host's immune response to its tumor is an
integrated series of complex events which is quite analogous to
a homo-transplantation reaction. However, it has been noted
that the host's immune response fails to eliminate its tumor
tissue (break in immune surveillance) and, in fact, as some investigators have postulated (12), may help in its growth. This
host immune reaction has been divided into three main compo-
nents--the afferent, central and efferent limbs--which are
described as follows:

The afferent limb is the inductive phase of the response and
includes the mechanisms by which antigenic tumor cells are

recognized and induce sensitization in the host.

The central limb concerns cell origin, diversity, recruitment, distribution and survival.

The efferent limb is responsible for final elimination (or stimulation) of the tumor cells by the effector mechanisms (cellular and/or humoral).

The effector cells (thymus-dependent cells?) in cellular response possess on their surface specific antigen receptors, which are triggered by contact with specific antigen. When such activated lymphocytes meet the cells carrying the activating antigen, this affects both the lymphocytes (by producing biologically active substances or transformation) and the target cells (by causing their destruction). This reaction lends itself to measurement in vitro (6).

The term "sensitized lymphocytes" denotes antigen reactive cells having receptors on their cell surface (probably produced by the cells, and similar to antibodies). These cells are instrumental in delayed type hypersensitivity and reactions similar to homograft rejection. In contrast, "cell mediated reaction" usually refers to a broader concept, irrespective of involvement of sensitized "lymphocytes" (preferably, lymphoid cells). The sensitized lymphocytes (effector cells) which can destroy cells carrying antigens (target cells) on contact are usually a heterogenous population of cells (mononuclear cells, macrophages, and polymorphonuclear cells) (13). This confusion, for practical purposes, can be minimized by stating in detail the conditions of each experiment.

Several in vitro and in vivo methods (Table 2) have recently been developed to identify those lymphoid cells in the host which are sensitized to its tumor or allograft. Most of these methods are

Table 2: Summary and principles of various in vivo and in vitro methods Used to assess sensitized lymphoid cells in tumor-host relationship (ref. reviews 6, 11, 13, 14, 36)

In vivo

1) Skin hypersensitivity test--Introduction of tumor antigens (soluble or killed tumor cells) in the skin of tumor-bearing host to elicit cutaneous delayed hypersensitivity reaction (32-35).

2) Neutralization test (review 6).

3) Transplantation technique (review 6).

In vitro

A. Target and lymphoid cell interaction

1) Destruction of monolayer (plaque technique).

2) Release of isotopes from specifically labeled target cells (such as ^{3}H or ^{14}C Thymidine, ^{32}P-Phosphate, ^{51}Cr-Chromate, etc.) in the presence of sensitized lymphoid cells.

3) Inhibition of isotope incorporation by target cells (radioactive thymidine).

4) Virus infection of sensitized lymphoid cells, i. e., virus plaque assay for antigen-sensitive cells in delayed hypersensitivity.

5) Inhibition of colony formation.

6) Macrophage migration and/or leucocyte migrations.

7) "Microcytotoxicity test", based on actual individual cell count in microtest plate (several modifications of this technique are presently in use in various laboratories).

8) "Mixed Lymphocyte Culture" technique.

B. Assays based on soluble factors (biologically active) produced by sensitized lymphocyte-target cell inter-action

1) Macrophage inhibition factor.

2) Lymphocyte transforming (blastogenic) factor.

3) Macrophage activating factor.

4) Monocyte chemotactic factor.

5) Skin reactive factor.

6) Lymphocyte cytotoxic factor.

7) Transfer factor.

based on sound principles and measure a specific aspect of the functions of these cells. But their experimental conditions and the interpretation of results obtained with them are not always ideal.

The goals of most of the methods used in tumor-host situations are threefold:

1. To provide a simplified in vitro system, a basis for under-standing and correlating the host in vivo immune responses to its tumor;

2. To identify the nature and cross reactivity of tumor-specific antigens;

3. To provide a reliable and useful in vitro test for assessment of immune responses due to various methods of immune manipu-lation, particularly when such assays can be applied to situations where in vivo testing is often not possible (clinical applications). PERLMAN and HOLM (13), BLOOM and GLADE (11), REVILLARD (14), OETTGEN and HELLSTRÖM (6), and OETTGEN and BEAN (36) have recently compiled critical sur-veys of many such methods introduced in the past decade.

We have used the modified microcytotoxicity test to study lymphocyte cytotoxicity in vitro and its correlation with status of tumor in vivo (2, 4). Furthermore, using the same techniques, we have investigated some facets of the antitumor immune responses (Immune Parameters, Table 3) in vitro and correlated them with tumor growth in vivo.

Table 3: Anti-tumor immune parameters

    1) Cell-Mediated Immunity

        a) Number of circulating lymphocytes.

        b) Quantitation of cytotoxicity on target cells by peripheral blood lymphocytes.

    2) Quantitation of Blocking Serum Factors in vitro.

    3) Quantitation of Cytotoxic Serum Activity in the Presence of: i) Rabbit Complement (xenogenic) and ii) W/Fu Rat Complement (homologous).

    4) Unblocking Serum Activity (capacity of sera to neutralize the blocking serum activity in vitro).

    5) Antibodies on Tumor Target Cells (in vivo)-- elution and biological characterization of tumor eluates in vitro and in vivo.

Some aspects of this technique and the results obtained by using this assay in the polyoma tumor-rat model will be discussed in detail.

Materials and Methods

The following is a general description of some problems that we have encountered in using methods based on lymphocyte-target cell interaction in vitro, and specific materials and methods used in the present study.

Microcytotoxicity test: This test is based on an actual count of target cells in the wells of the microtest plate (3040 II). It has largely replaced the original Colony Inhibition test and gives results similar to that of Colony Inhibition (see review 11).

Selection of target cells for seeding in microwells: The moderately overgrown monolayer of polyoma tumor cell culture is trypsinized (1:250 trypsin solution) 1-2 days prior to experiment; half the cell suspension is passaged to obtain a monolayer culture of target cells. On the day of experiment the culture should be in monolayer . (If bottles contain areas of overgrowth, coarse granulation in the cells, too many dead floating cells in the supernatant, different morphology (large ghost cells) in different areas of the monolayer, extremely acidic pH of the culture media, etc., this is an indication of poor selection of cells). On the day of experiment the supernatant from the bottle is discarded and remaining medium is washed either with plain EAGLE's medium or half-strength trypsin solution. Then one to two ml of trypsin is added to the bottle and the bottle is incubated at 37°C for two-three minutes. The monolayer is brought into single cell suspension by gentle shaking at the end of incubation period, and the trypsin effect is immediately neutralized by adding WAYMOUTH medium containing 20% foetal calf serum. The cell suspension is examined under inverted microscope; if there are too many clumps of cells present in the suspension, the bottle is discarded. Only suspensions having single cells are used. The viability of cells is checked by the dye exclusion test (21). Suspensions containing 95% or more viable cells are used for seeding in the microtest plate. Figure 1 summarizes the test performed for quantitation of lymphocyte cytotoxicity in the rat-polyoma model. The test for blocking serum factors

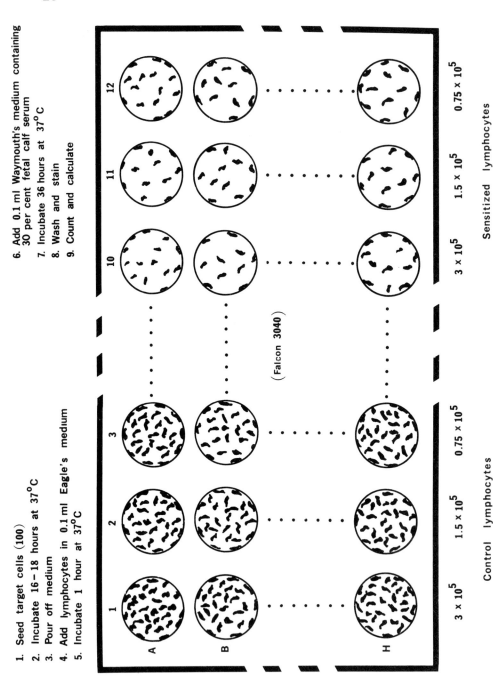

Fig. 1. Diagramatic presentation of lymphocyte cytotoxic test

has been described elsewhere (11, 15).

The cell concentration is adjusted (in WAYMOUTH medium containing 20% foetal calf serum) so that each 0.2 ml contains 100 viable cells. The cells are then seeded by inoculating 0.2 ml of cell suspension in each well with a 0.2 ml pipette. The speed and accuracy with which cells are inoculated are important.

<u>Experimental steps:</u> The microplates are incubated in a CO_2 incubator at $37^{\circ}C$ for 16-18 hours. At the end of that time the plates are examined for:

1. Morphology and number of cells in each well;
2. Clumping of colonies of cells (if several colonies of cells are seen, the plates are discarded).

If the number of cells is too great or too small (ideal is 70-80 cells per well), or if the morphology is not satisfactory (granulation or round cells), one of the plates is stained with crystal violet and the remaining attached cells are counted in approximately 20 wells. If the plates are considered to be satisfactory (with respect to cell count, distribution and morphology), the experiment proceeds as outlined in Figure 1.

In this method the remaining individual living attached cells are counted. The final cell count may be influenced by:

1. Target cell proliferation;
2. Some toxic material or uneven surface of the microtest plate;
3. Period of lymphocyte-target cell interaction;
4. Feeder or toxic effect of lymphocytes (depends upon number of lymphocytes-- a small number gives feeder effect);
5. Toxic or feeder effect of sera or medium;
6. Toxic and stimulating effect of cell metabolites (conditioning of tissue culture medium-- produced during incubation);

7. Non-immune allogenic effect;

8. In vitro sensitization of non-sensitized lymphocytes;

9. Uneven pH in the different wells;

10. Sensitivity of different target cells;

11. Error in counting of remaining cells;

12. Inappropriate control;

13. Different serum concentrations in control and test wells;

14. Contamination in plate;

15. Too vigorous or slow stirring of cell suspension solution when seeding;

16. Inappropriate seeding in microwells.

Most of these problems can be well controlled by:

1. Keeping source of material constant;

2. Maintaining a constant environment for each successive experiment;

3. Knowing the growth behavior and plating efficiency of the target cells;

4. Performing criss-cross controls (16, 17); and

5. Using enough replicates for each test.

Furthermore, some of the drawbacks can be circumvented by performing vertical studies (17, 18) on the same experimental animal.

Target cells: Several kinds of cultivated cells in different types of medium enriched with sera from different sources have been utilized. Both established cell lines and primary cell cultures, each of which has certain advantages and disadvantages, are used. In the former, the cells are adapted to specific culture conditions and are sources of stable, sensitive target cells for each successive experiment. But such lines may get infected with viruses or mycoplasma, thus acquiring new antigens or losing existing ones. On the other hand, short primary cultures have the disadvantage of having a heterogenous population of cells and being more sensitive to changes of tissue culture media. It seems that the actual sensitivity of cells to the cytotoxic effect of lymphocytes or antibody and complement is probably controlled by many factors besides the concentration of antigenic sites on the surface of the cells (see page 1158, ref. 25). It has been argued by some investigators (36) that cells obtained from a fresh tumor tissue specimen are the only true representative of the tumor in vivo. It is also argued that the use of enzymes to obtain cell suspension may alter the antigens on the cell surface. However, it can be counter-argued that cells obtained from fresh tumor may have antibodies absorbed on their cell surface, which may interfere with the in vitro test (17). Furthermore, it is not always technically possible to have a good suspension of living cells from tumor tissue by mechnical means alone. Such cell suspensions may be contaminated with lymphocytes or macrophages from the tumor tissue.

In our own work, we have used primary cultures of Polyoma 20 (PW-20) and Polyoma 21 (PW-21), which will be described (infra), and Polyoma 13 (PW-13), which has been described previously (18). The cell cultures were renewed after 15-20 serial passages in tissue cultures by explanting tumor carried in vivo in syngeneic animals or from cells (8-11 generations) frozen in liquid nitrogen. The culture conditions were kept constant and tissue culture media were prepared weekly from stock solutions. The concentration of foetal calf sera was kept constant for each type of cell line during cultivation and experimentation. Optimal number of cells needed for seeding to obtain 60-70% plating efficiency was calculated for each type of tumor target cells. Such efforts are important in order to minimize some of the problems associated with the use of primary cultures in this technique.

Separation of lymphocytes: Several techniques are available for the separation of various types of cells from blood, spleen and lymphnode cell suspensions. The cytotoxic effect of the lymphocyte suspension may be influenced by the method of its preparation (36). These methods are based on the differences in the specific gravity of the cells, roulex formation, chemical differences or varying electrophoretic mobility. The technique we have used was described by PERTOFF et al. (19). Separation of lymphocytes from blood was accomplished by centrifugation on density cushions of silica gel. Lymphocytes were obtained in a narrow band in the interphase between cushions having a density of 1.0770 and 1.0500. They were sucked off, washed with EAGLE's medium, incubated with glutathione, washed a second time with the same medium, spun down, counted and used in the cytotoxicity test. Blood was obtained from the femoral vein of an experimental rat in a heparinized syringe. This technique gives a high yield (> 80%) of pure lymphocytes even with small volumes (1.0 ml) of blood; furthermore, the cell suspension is very minimally contaminated with red blood cells, polymorphonuclear cells and platelets (less than 2-3%). But when the test animals are carrying large tumor load, have ulcerated, infected subcutaneous tumors, or are clinically uraemic and quite sick, the contamination of red blood cells and polymorphs is usually higher. Even minute blood clots in the specimen may lead to higher contamination and poor yield. The viability of cells is usually over 98% and the cells are reactive in vitro (SJÖGREN and

BANSAL, unpublished findings). Thus, this technique is considered quite suitable for use in the present study.

The contamination with red blood cells (free hemoglobulin) and polymorphonuclear cells may affect the in vitro results in this and many of the other assay systems mentioned. The preparations of lymphocytes obtained by this technique are not contaminated with clumps of platelets and thus do not exhibit non-specific toxicity as sometimes seen in lymphocytes obtained by the ficol-hypaque technique (35).

Animals and tumors: Rats of the inbred (brother mated to sister) W/Fu strain were used. Their origin and maintenance have been discussed previously (18). These rats accept skin grafts from each other permanently and reject a foreign skin graft (from inbred B/N rats) in the normal fashion (20).

Primary kidney and skin sarcomas were induced by subcutaneous inoculation of polyoma virus in newborn W/Fu rats (4). Polyoma tumor 13 (PW-13) was used for most of the in vivo and in vitro experiments. Histologically, this tumor, along with Polyoma 20 (PW-20) and Polyoma 21 (PW-21), is a fibrosarcoma. PW-13 is highly anaplastic in character; PW-20 is relatively scirrhous and has a firm gritty feeling to a cut surface; PW-21 is a very firm, cartilagenous tumor. Tumors induced by polyoma virus have common tumor-specific antigens. This was demonstrated by the fact that lymphocytes from a rat bearing one of these three types of polyoma tumor exerted a cytotoxic effect on the target cells derived from any of these tumor cell lines. However, when testing for blocking of cytotoxic effect of sensitized lymphocytes by serum factors, additional and somewhat different information was obtained: the sera from rats bearing

one type of polyoma tumor (PW-13) abrogated the cytotoxic effect of sensitized lymphocytes best in the specific lymphocyte-
target cell combination (PW-13) as compared to different lymphocyte-target cell combinations (PW-21). Furthermore, in
certain lymphocyte (PW-20)-target cell (PW-21) combinations,
either barely significant or no blocking activity could be obtained
by testing with serum from another polyoma-bearing rat (PW-13).
This suggests that tumors induced by polyoma virus may have
individual tumor-specific antigens, in addition to common tumor-
specific antigens described previously (BANSAL and SJÖGREN,
unpublished findings). It may prove to be very important, when
studying human tumors (having cross-reacting tumor antigens),
to make an appropriate selection of lymphocyte-target cell combinations, particularly when testing for blocking effect on the
sensitized lymphocytes by serum factors.

Viability of cells: The viability of cells was checked by the
trypan blue exclusion test (21).

Tumor volume: The tumor volume was calculated by the technique described by ATTIA et al. (22).

Complement: Homologous complement (W/Fu) was obtained
from a pool of animals used for each successive experiment
performed. The technique of collecting complement is described
elsewhere (4).

In order to obtain xenogenic complement, a number of rabbits
were bled and serum from each rabbit was tested on polyoma
target cells for non-specific sera toxicity. The rabbits showing
insignificant (less than 10%) toxicity were used as donors of
rabbit complement.

BCG: Viable organisms (0, 6 mg/ml) obtained by suspending freeze dried vaccine (Research Foundation, Chicago, Illinois) in saline were used.

Anti-lymphocyte sera (A. L. S. -antirat-rabbit): ALS was prepared as described by LEVEY and MEDAWAR (23).

Elution of antibodies from tumor tissue: The technique of eluting antibodies from tumor tissue (in vivo) has been described elsewhere (18).

Correlation of in vitro and in vivo findings: The technique described above affords the opportunity for analysis of various immune responses in small animals. We made "vertical analyses", i. e. , the same animal was studied at different time points, with respect to cellular and humoral responses in vitro and the results were correlated with the status of its tumor in vivo. The effects due to immune manipulation (such as BCG inoculation, ALS treatment, unblocking serum therapy, surgery, etc.) in the tumor-bearing host were also studied. Such in vitro studies done in the same experimental animal under stable conditions circumvent or minimize some of the problems encountered with this technique. This type of in vitro analysis and correlation of the results obtained with the in vivo situation of the tumor-bearing host is analogous to the problem of studying a similar situation in tumor-bearing humans.

Results and Discussion

Effect of tumor mass, excision of tumor, and regional and pulmonary metastasis on the quantitative cytotoxic effect of sensitized lymphocytes: We earlier concluded (3) from our studies that there is no major breakdown of cell-mediated immunity in polyoma-bearing W/Fu rats at various time points during the progressive growth of their tumor. By studying the cytotoxic effect of a fixed number of blood lymphocytes, we also concluded that there is no significant difference in cell-mediated immunity between experimental rats bearing progressively growing tumors of different sizes and rats which have had their tumors excised. However, when studies were done by serial dilution of lymphocytes to find the minimum number of lymphocytes needed to obtain a significant cytotoxic effect on tumor target cells, a correlation between cytotoxic effect of lymphocytes in vitro and tumor growth in vivo was found (Table 4, ref. 17).

We did not find any correlation between number of circulating lymphocytes in the host and growth of its tumor in vivo (17). This is in contrast to the findings of RIESCO (24), who reported a significant correlation between this parameter of existing immune response and cancer curability in humans.

Effect of BCG and ALS (Antilymphocyte serum) therapy on cytotoxic effect of sensitized lymphocytes: It has been demonstrated that non-specific stimulation of the host with BCG prior to tumor isograft usually causes tumor inhibition (26-28). We have studied the quantitative changes in the cytotoxic effect of blood lymphocytes from rats treated with BCG in this model (Figure 2, detail published elsewhere, 29). Our results indicate that a single dose of BCG given two weeks prior or on the day of tumor isograft causes a moderate inhibition of tumor growth(29). Using the microcytotoxicity test, we also demonstrated a significant increase in the cytotoxic effect of sensitized lymphocytes from rats treated with BCG (Figure 2 and ref. 29). However, if the BCG was given after tumor had already appeared, neither tumor inhibition in vivo nor increase in the cytotoxic effect of host's blood lymphocytes in vitro was detected (29).

Table 4: Summary of information obtained in polyoma-rat model, correlation between sensitized lymphocyte activity in vitro and status of tumor in vivo

Time in Days	Status of tumor in vivo	Number of test lymphocytes as compared to control lymphocytes			
		3×10^5	1.5×10^5	0.75×10^5	0.37×10^5
0-3	Isograft of 2×10^6 PW-13 cells in flank (induction period)	−	−	−	−
4-7	Tumor not palpable (induction period)	+	+	+/−	−
7-14	Small tumor (0.5-1.5 cms)(early growth)	+	+	+/−	−
14-21	Large tumor (>2.0 cms)(late growth)	+	+	+/−	−
21-35	Large tumor (>3.0 cms) with regional lymphnode and distant metastasis	+	+/−	−	−
0-184	After excision of tumor isograft and rat is clinically free of tumor	+	+	+/−	−
0-7	After excision of tumor isograft and regional lymphnodes, but residual tumor in the lungs	+	+/−	+/−	−
> 7	As above	+	+/−	−	−

+ Significant cytotoxic effect in all rats tested
+/− Some of the rats tested had significant effect
− None of the rats tested had significant effect

Lymphocyte cytotoxicity indicates target cells killed after exposure to test lymphocytes as compared to the same number of control lymphocytes. The probability that the differences are significant was calculated by Student's test.

Furthermore, BCG given in the latter situation caused significant enhanced tumor growth, which has been attributed to blocking serum factors (29). The foregoing emphasizes that administration of BCG may have different effects on antitumor immune
responses of the host depending upon: 1)type and dose of BCG;
2) immune status of the host at the time of BCG therapy. This
indicates that the various host immune parameters listed in
Table 3 should be analyzed in vitro prior to and during the BCG
therapy (30).

Patients treated with sufficient doses of antilymphocyte serum
(ALS) exhibited impaired cutaneous hypersensitivity reactions,
and the lymphocytes from such patients showed decreased stim-
ulation (in vitro) with different antigens. It was concluded that
ALS induces a split defect of cell-mediated immunity (see
REVILLARD in ref. 14, page 174).

We have studied the in vitro cytotoxic effect on tumor-bearing
rats treated with ALS immediately prior to tumor isograft. Our

Fig. 2. Effect of BCG and ALS therapy on sensitized lymphocytes

---

Group I-Control; Group II-0.1 ml of BCG inoculated intracutane-
ously (I.C.) on the opposite flank on the day of tumor isograft;
Group III-0.1 ml of BCG inoculated I.C. 2 weeks prior to tumor
isograft; Group IV-rats received 0.5 ml of ALS intraperitoneally
7 days prior to and on the day of isografting.
    Insuf. Lymph. (Insufficient number lymphocytes on separa-
    tion from blood samples for the exp.) . Percent cytotoxicity
    is calculated by comparing the reduction of cells, by sensi-
    tized lymphocytes as compared to equal number of control
    lymphocytes.
    Numbers indicated are number of lymphocytes/ml of blood
    x 10^6 on the day of experiment; the number indicated above
    each bar is the number of lymphocytes x 10^5 used in each
    well.

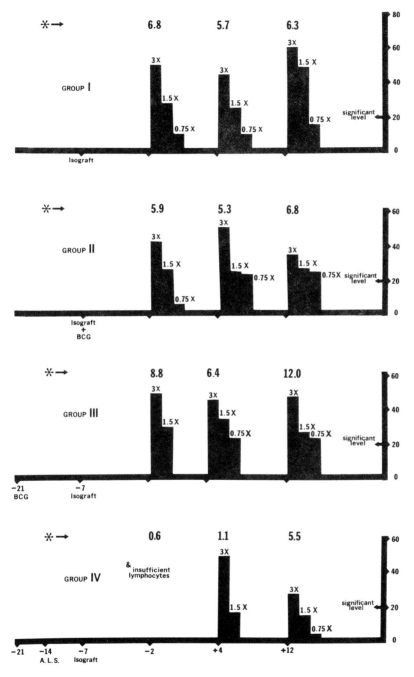

✳→ 6.8 5.7 6.3

GROUP I

3 X
1.5 X
0.75 X
significant level

Isograft

✳→ 5.9 5.3 6.8

GROUP II

3 X
1.5 X
0.75 X
significant level

Isograft
+
BCG

✳→ 8.8 6.4 12.0

GROUP III

3 X
1.5 X
0.75 X
significant level

−21 −7
BCG Isograft

✳→ 0.6 1.1 5.5

GROUP IV

& insufficient
lymphocytes

3 X
1.5 X
0.75 X
significant level

−21 −14 −7 −2 +4 +12
A.L.S. Isograft

Time in Days in Relation to Tumor Appearance

⁺Percent Cytotoxicity with Indicated Number x 10⁵ Lymphocytes

results indicate a significant decrease in the cytotoxic effect of
peripheral sensitized lymphocytes in vitro and enhanced tumor
growth in vivo (29). However, the lymphocytes from tumor-
bearing host treated with ALS were capable of exerting a cytotoxic effect on specific target cells in vitro (Figure 2 and ref.
29).

Up to this point, I have discussed some of the problems with
respect to the techniques and information obtained in identifying
the tumor sensitized lymphocytes in a variety of situations, by
using the microcytotoxicity test. Using the same in vitro technique, HELLSTRÖMS and others (2, 3) have demonstrated that
factors that can specifically block the cytotoxic effects of immune lymphocytes are regularly demonstrable in the serum of
various experimental animals and human patients carrying a
tumor. The time of appearance in the serum and significance of
these blocking serum factors have been studied in the rat-polyoma model (17). Serum blocking factors could be detected more
than one week prior to a palpable tumor mass in most rats
which developed primary neoplasms after polyoma virus infection as newborns (30, 31). In all of these test rats, sensitized
lymphocytes could also be demonstrated in vitro. In this tumor
system, the titre of blocking activity increased rapidly and
reached its maximum level when tumor was clinically palpable
(4). This blocking activity was maintained until the rat died (4).
Similarly, in rats which were given polyoma isograft, the blocking activity appeared in the serum of most animals one or two
days prior to actual palpation of tumor nodule (18). We found
that this blocking activity is absorbed onto tumor tissue in vivo
and can be eluted by low pH treatment (18); such tumor eluates
have blocking activity in vitro (18); and inoculation of blocking

serum factors and tumor eluate causes tumor enhancement in
vivo. Some of the main findings from our model are summarized
in Table 5.

Table 5: Summary of some important findings obtained in
polyoma-rat model

Rat with Tumor	Test	Same Rat Tested 7 Days After Tumor Excision
+	Cytotoxic lymphocytes	+
+	Serum blocking in vitro	-
+	Serum from rat--capable of enhancing growth of polyoma tumor isograft	-
+	Cytotoxic serum activity in the presence of rabbit complement	+
-	Cytotoxic serum activity in the presence of rat (homologous)complement	+
-	Unblocking serum activity	$\pm$
+	"Probability" of take of small polyoma tumor test graft	-

+ indicates positive in all tested animals
+ indicates positive in some of the animals tested
$\overline{-}$ indicates negative in all tested animals

The present model has afforded evidence of a subtle balance between antitumor immunity capable of causing tumor rejection

and factors in the serum which can abrogate this effect, as shown below:

Cell-mediated immunity
(sensitized lymphocytes,
other mechanisms)   Blocking serum factors

+   +

Cytotoxic and unblocking   ⇌   Antibodies on target
serum factors   cells

+   +

Unknown   Unknown

Several in vitro techniques now are available to analyze these various facets of antitumor immune responses. Many of the in vitro techniques mentioned have already been put to use in clini-

Table 6: In vitro methods and their possible in vivo correlates

stage of response in vivo	possible in vitro methods to study
Antigen priming ⟶	Lymphocyte stimulation by antigen
Antigen recognition ⟶	Rosette formation test
Antigen processing ⟶	HOLM's test (1969).
Immune response ⟶	
Antibody formation ⟶	1. Local haemolysis test 2. Microcytotoxicity test 3. Others
Cellular response	
Delayed hypersensitivity⟶	1. Macrophage migration inhibition 2. Lymphocyte stimulation by antigen?
Effector cells (Sensitized lymphocytes) ⟶	1. Colony Inhibition 2. Microcytotoxicity test 3. Isotope release 4. Inhibition of radioactive isotopes by target cells 5. Biologically active mediators

cal problems. But if the data obtained is to form a basis for future clinical application, a rigorous attempt must be made to
study different phases of immune responses by a variety of in
vitro methods in the same test animal. Table 6 summarizes a
few of these in vitro methods and their possible in vivo counter-
parts (13, 14). These represent successive stages from antigen
priming of, and recognition by, antigen sensitive cells to their
expression as sensitized lymphocytes.

Summary

Recent information indicates that both experimental tumors in
animals and spontaneous tumors in humans exhibit weak antigenic responses in the host of origin. A specific antitumor immune response against tumor-specific (associated) antigens has
been demonstrated by the presence of sensitized lymphoid cells
and humoral antibodies in the tumor-bearing host.

This paper summarizes several facets of problems encountered
in studies concerning the presence of sensitized lymphocytes in
a polyoma-rat model. In these studies the modified microcytotoxicity test was used. It is based on the measurement of tumor
target cell destruction following lymphocyte-target cell interaction in vitro. The cytotoxicity of lymphocytes from sensitized
donors, which was demonstrated by this method, has been assumed to be an in vitro manifestation of delayed hypersensitivity
and similar phenomena in vivo. However, this assumption may
not hold for all situations.

Furthermore, the paper describes the effect of BCG and antilymphocyte therapy on sensitized lymphocytes in the tumor-
bearing host.

Acknowledgement

Part of the work presented here has been published in detail elsewhere. This work was done in the laboratories of Prof. Hans O. SJÖGREN and Profs. K. E. and I. HELLSTRÖM in Seattle, Washington.

The author gratefully acknowledges the kindness of Prof. K. E. HELLSTRÖM, Department of Pathology, University of Washington, Seattle, Washington, and Prof. D. HUME and Prof. H. M. LEE, Department of Surgery, Medical College of Virginia, Richmond, Virginia, for making critical comments in the preparation of this manuscript.

The skillful technical assistance of Mr. Richard HARGREAVES and Miss Carol DUNSMOOR, is also gratefully acknowledged.

This investigation was supported by Grants CA10188, CA10189 and CA11742 from the National Institutes of Health, by Grant T-453 from the American Cancer Society, and by Contract NIH-NCI-71-2171 within the Special Virus Cancer Program of the NIH.

References

1. HELLSTRÖM, K. E. & HELLSTRÖM, I. (1970), Ann. Rev. Microbiol. 24, 373.

2. HELLSTRÖM, K. E. & HELLSTRÖM, I. (1969), Adv. Cancer Res. 12, 167.

3. SJÖGREN, H. O. & BANSAL, S. C. (1972), Antigens in virally induced tumors, in Progress in Immunology (ed. Amos, B.), Academic Press, New York.

4. BANSAL, S. C. & SJÖGREN, H. O. (1972), Int. J. Cancer 9, 490.

5. POLLOCK, S., Specific "arming" of normal lymphnode cells by sera from tumor bearing mice. Int. J. Cancer (to be published).

6. OETTGEN, H. F. & HELLSTRÖM, K. E. (1973), Tumor Immunology, in Cancer Medicine (ed. Frei, E. & Holland, J.).

7. McKHANN, C. F. & JAGARLAMOODY, M. (1972), Evidence for immune reactivity against neoplasms, in Transplantation Review (ed. Moller, G.), vol. 7, The Williams & Wilkins Company, U.S.A.

8. SJÖGREN, H. O. (1965), Progr. Exp. Tumor Res. 6, 289.

9. KLEIN, G. (1971), Israel J. Med. Sci. 7, 111.

10. MORTON, D. L. (1972), Cancer 30, 1647.

11. BLOOM, B. R. & GLADE, P. R., eds. (1971), In vitro Methods in Cell-Mediated Immunity, Academic Press, New York.

12. PREHN, R. T. & LAPPE, M. A. (1971), An immunostimulation theory of tumor development, in Transplantation Review (ed. Moller, G.), vol. 7, The Williams & Wilkins Company.

13. PERLMAN, P. & HOLM, G. (1969), Adv. Immunology 11, 117.

14. REVILLARD, J. P., ed. (1971), Cell Mediated Immunity in vitro Correlates, University Park Press, U.S.A.

15. BANSAL, S. C. & SJÖGREN, H. O., In vitro testing of enhancement, Transplantation Proc. (in press).

16. HELLSTRÖM, K. E. & HELLSTRÖM, I., The role of cell-mediated immunity in control of tumors, in Immunobiology (eds. Bach, F. & Good, R. A.) (in press).

17. BANSAL, S. C. & SJÖGREN, H. O., Correlation between changes in antitumor immune parameters and tumor growth in vivo in rats, Fed. Proc. (in press).

18. BANSAL, S. C. & SJÖGREN, H. O. (1972), Int. J. Cancer 9, 97.

19. PERTOFF, H., BOCK, O. & LINDAHL-KIESSLING, K. (1968), Exp. Cell Res. 50, 355.

20. BANSAL, S. C., HELLSTRÖM, K. E., HELLSTRÖM, I. & SJÖGREN, H. O., Cell-mediated immunity and blocking serum activity to tolerated allografts in rats, J. Exp. Med. (in press).

21. BOYSE, E. A., OLD, L. J. & THOMAS, G. (1962), Transplantation Bull. 29, 63.

22. ATTIA, M. A., DeOME, K. B. & WEISS, D. W. (1965), Cancer Res. 25, 451.

23. LEVEY, R.H. & MEDAWAR, P.B. (1966), Ann. N.Y. Acad. Sci. 129, 164.

24. RIESCO, A. (1970), Cancer 25, 135.

25. McKHANN, C.F. (1971), Transplantation Proc. 3, 1158.

26. WEISS, D.W., BONHAG, R.S. & DeOME, K.B. (1966), Nature (London) 190, 889.

27. WEISS, D.W., BONHAG, R.S. & LESLIE, P. (1966), J. Exp. Med. 124, 1039.

28. OLD, L.J., BENACERRAF, B., CLARKE, D.A., CARSWELL, E.A. & STOCKERT, E. (1961), Cancer Res. 21, 1281.

29. BANSAL, S.C. & SJÖGREN, H.O., Effects of BCG on various facets of immune response against polyoma tumors in rats, Int. J. Cancer (in press).

30. BANSAL, S.C. & SJÖGREN, H.O., Regression of polyoma tumor metastasis by combined unblocking and BCG treatment. -Correlation with induced alterations in tumor immunity status, Int. J. Cancer (to be submitted).

31. SJÖGREN, H.O. & BORUM, K. (1971), Cancer Res. 31, 890.

32. OETTGEN, H.F., OLD, L.J., McLEAN, E.P. & CARSWELL, E.A. (1968), Nature (London) 220, 295.

33. CHURCHILL, W.H., RAPP, H., KRONMAN, B.S. & BORSOS, T. (1968), J. Nat. Cancer Inst. 41, 13.

34. HUGHES, I.F. & LYTTON, B. (1964), Brit. Med. J. 1, 209.

35. STEWART, T.H.M. (1969), Cancer 23, 1368.

36. OETTGEN, H.F. & BEAN, M.A. (1972), Cancer Res. 32, 2845.

1.3 The Mixed Lymphocyte Tumor Cell Culture (MLTC) Test: Review of a Method

G. A. Nagel, E. Nagel, R. Albrecht and E. L. Bauder

Lymphocytes are of the major cell populations of the surveillance system which governs immunological host defense mechanisms. Lymphocytes are easily cultured and their in vitro response to antigens correlates to a large extent to the lymphocyte donor's immune status. The development of small lymphocytes into large blast-like cells and mitoses in vitro is known as lymphocyte transformation, lymphocyte stimulation or lymphocyte blastogenesis. The morphological changes or the extent of DNA which is freshly synthesized during the transformation process generally serve as parameters to determine the degree of lymphocyte reactivity in vitro.

Substances which induce lymphocyte transformation in vitro are called stimulants or mitogens and might be classified into two main groups: 1)Non-specific mitogens such as phytohemagglutinin (PHA), Pokeweed mitogen, bacterial products, UV-light, etc.; 2)Specific mitogens, i.e. substances mostly of antigenic character such as penicillin, tuberculin, viruses, Candidin, etc., to which the lymphocyte donor has been previously sensitized (1).

Cells or cellular components might act as specific mitogens too. Thus BAIN et al. (2) showed transformation of lymphocytes in the presence of allogeneic leukocytes. This finding has been

[1] Supported by Grant No. FOR. 025. AK. 72 (1)from Swiss Cancer League

confirmed by others and is thought to be a model for the recognition phase of the homograft rejection (3). Lymphocyte transformation, however, is not confined to stimulation by cells allogeneic to the lymphocyte donor but is also found with cells of autochthonous origin, for instance autologous platelets in patients with idiopathic thrombocytopenic purpura (4). This type of lymphocyte reactivity might be looked at as autoimmune reaction in vitro.

Since at the present time there is suggesting evidence that membranes of cancer cells bear antigens foreign to the cancer patient's normal cell population the question was raised whether the lymphocyte culture system might be a tool to reflect the existence of antigenic differences between host and tumor. In fact several authors reported blastogenic response of lymphocytes to extracts or homogenates of tumor cells (5, 6) or to viable tumor cells (7, 8, 9, 10, 11). Accordingsly the MLTC test appears to be a promising technique for further studies in immune oncology.

The MLTC test, however, is far from being standardized. The method varies considerably from one laboratory to another. Moreover numerous factors which influence the outcome of the MLTC are poorly understood and difficult to control. We have therefore concentrated our efforts on the establishment of the optimal in vitro conditions needed to study this type of lymphocyte-tumor cell interaction and hereby present what has been the best method in our hands.

The method

Lymphocytes

Lymphocytes are obtained essentially by the method of BÖYUM (12). 20 ml of venous blood is drawn into a plastic syringe containing 1 ml of heparin (1000 U/ml) free of preservatives and carefully layered on to 12 ml of an aquaeus solution of 9% Ficoll-34% Ronpacon (24:10, density 1.077) in 50 ml thick walled centrifuge glass tubes. The gradients are centrifuged at 1400 g for 10 min. during which the granulocytes and red cells sediment through the Ficoll-Ronpacon phase. Lymphocytes forming a layer at the interphase between the plasma and the Ficoll-Ronpacon mixtures are collected by aspiration into a siliconised glass centrifuge tube, washed twice in MEM-EAGLE medium (with 2000 i.U. of penicillin and 0.1 mg streptomycin but without serum). Cells are centrifuged at 700 g for the first and 250 g for the second washing. Lymphocytes are resuspended in 2 ml of MEM and counted with 1% acetic acid in a hemocytometer. Viability is assessed by trypan blue exclusion. With this isolation technique lymphocyte viability usually is 100% and contamination with non-mononuclear cells always less than 5%. For differential counts a smear is made and dyed with GIEMSA stain.

Tumor cells

Tumors from biopsies or operation specimens are obtained directly from the operating room and processed within 10-30 min. after removal. They are cut into small pieces of approximatively 1 mm^3 with forceps, scissors or knife, put into 15 ml of MEM + antibiotics as mentioned above + 0.25% cristallinized trypsin (Difco) and carefully stirred with a magnetic stirrer at room temperature. The supernatant is decanted into a 20 ml glass centrifuge tube as soon as it looks turbid (after 5-10 min.) and replaced by 15 ml of fresh trypsin solution. This procedure is repeated several times until the supernatant remains clear. Trypsinization never should exceed 45 min.

The tumor cells are washed three times in MEM + antibiotics and centrifuged at 200 g for 5 min. at room temperature and resuspended in 2-4 ml MEM depending on the number of cells.

Alternatively tumor cells are obtained as cell suspension from carcinomatous exsudates. Such cells are either immediately washed or if heavily contaminated by red cells purified on a Ficoll-Ronpacon gradient as mentioned above. Viability testing is done by the trypan blue test.

MLTC

The medium used for culture is MEM-EAGLE medium as described above with 10% pooled heat inactivated human AB-serum added. Lymphocyte concentration is adjusted to 1×10^6/ml and tumor cell concentration to 5×10^6 and 0.2×10^6 viable cells per ml. Within each experiment the number of responding lymphocytes is kept constant at 0.5×10^6 cells per culture tube; tumor cells are added in numbers to make final lymphocyte: tumor cell ratios of 1:1, 5:1, 25:1, 50:1. The final volume per tube is 1 ml. For culture we use Falcon plastic tubes 12 x 75 mm with snap closing lids. Each experiment is done in triplicate with the patient's own lymphocytes and with the lymphocytes of a normal control donor.

MLTC with lymphocytes and tumor cells deriving from the same cell donor are called autologous cultures in contrast to homologous cultures which are mixtures of lymphocytes and tumor cells deriving from different patients.

Culture labelling and counting

The tubes are closed and kept at 37° in static upright position for 5 days. For the last 16-18 hours of the culture period 50 λ 3H-thymidin (specific activity 5 Ci/mmol., 0.5 μCi/5 λ) are

added to each tube. The experiments are terminated by precipitation with 10% ice-cold trichlor-acetic acid (TCA) in a glass
tube of 100 x 15 mm, centrifugation for 10 min. at 250 g at 4°,
decanting, and drying off the rim of the culture tube with absorb-
ent paper towel. After having been shaken vigorously the samples
are washed twice with ice-cold TCA 5% and centrifuged for 10
min. at 250 g. The pellet is then dehydrated with cold aethanol
and centrifuged for 10 min. at 800 g. This pellet remains
unshaken. 0.5 ml soluene and as soon as the supernatant is
clear 0.025 ml distilled water is added to reduce quenching. 10
ml toluol-PPO-POPOP-solution (13) is filled into the tubes and
the samples are put into plastic scintillation counter bottles and
counted for 10 min.in a PICKER-scintillation counter. Results
are expressed in cpm.

Controls

Since many unspecific factors may either stimulatory or inhibitory interfere with lymphocyt e DNA-synthesis in vitro a wide
spectrum of controls is required. Therefore the following controls should be done whenever possible.

To test for "spontaneous" transformation the following cell
preparations are cultured alone without further mitogen added
in a concentration of 0.5×10^6 and 1×10^6 cells per tube.
Lymphocytes; mitomycin C treated lymphocytes" stimulating
cells (lymphocytes or tumor cells) with and without mitomycin
C treatment.

To control for viability and the ability of lymphocytes to respond to soluble stimuli: responding cells and stimulating cells
each with or without mitomycin C treatment in separate cultures
stimulated by PHA.

To control for the ability of lymphocytes to respond to cellular antigens a mixed one way lymphocyte culture (3) is done with stimulating mitomycin C lymphocytes from a lymphocyte pool stored at -170°.

To exclude the possibility that the stimulating cell population itself accounts for DNA-synthesis in addition to the above mentioned controls a mixture is set up with tumor cells and mitomycin C treated autologous or homologous lymphocytes.

To test whether lymphocyte transformation in the presence of autochthonous tumor cells is not a tumor-specific phenomenon but rather related to unspecific factors such as cell crowding a mixed culture with lymphocytes and normal tissue cells histologically similar to the tumor is advisable.

Replicate culture of the above mentioned MLTC and controls might be harvested on different days between the third and tenth culture day not to miss the day of maximal DNA-synthesis.

Further controls for inhibitory factors within the culture serum, bacterial contamination of the cultures, etc. are done when indicated.

Discussion

Working with the above described method several problems have to be dealt with. First of all we use exclusively fresh tumor cells and no cells from cultured cell lines. This is done because long-term cultures may change the antigenic properties of cells (14). Furthermore viable cells are thought to be more apt to induce blastogenesis than desintegrating or dead cells that may have lost part ot their antigens or membrane properties essential for induction of stimulation (11). Utmost precautions therefore are taken to damage tumor cells as little as possible.

The time of processing tumor and tumor cells is kept short; it is essential that tumors are processed immediately after surgical removal. To supply adequate nutrition tumor pieces and cells are kept in tissue culture medium throughout the different steps of the experiment.

Frequently isolation of the cells by trypsinization is superior to mechanical means. After our experience isolation of cells from the same tumor by mechanical means (scissors, forceps, knive and sieve) yields the same amount of cells when compared to enzymatic isolation but a percentage up to ten times higher will be dead. In addition very fibrous tumors are difficult to process mechanically only. Sometimes good results with trypsin-separation until the tumor material gets softer and then pressing material through a fine mesh gauze into a funnel are obtained.

Occasionally cell suspensions have a tendency to form fibrous aggregates where the isolated cells get entangled. With 1-2 drops DNAse per 2 ml (80 Kunitz U/ml) this mucoid material can easily be dispersed.

To avoid further mechanical damage to the separated cells centrifugation time is kept short and g as low as possible. Each sample is washed immediately after having been decanted from trypsinization; to further reduce the activity of the remaining trypsin medium and centrifuge are cooled to $4^{\circ}C$. Trypsin activity is never neutralized by addition of serum nor is serum added to the medium prior to cell counting since serum is known to lead to false positive viability values if they are assessed by trypan blue exclusion.

Freshly isolated cells seem to be extremely fragile. We therefore frequently keep our cells in medium + 5-10% serum overnight to give the cells that are able to recover and others that
are in the process of desintegration time to do so. Thus cell
viability sometimes is higher the morning after separation.
Mitomycin C treatment for DNA inhibition might further damage
freshly isolated cells and thereby reduce their blastogenic activity. Since in pilot studies we found that under the culture conditions mentioned above tumor cells are usually not able to synthesize DNA to any critical extent neither treatment with
mitomycin C nor with irradiation is done anymore.

Pooled human AB-serum that had been inactivated for 60 min.
at 56°C is chosen because fetal calf serum frequently stimulates
lymphocytes. Autologous patient serum is not used in order to
prevent introduction of additional unknown factors such as enhancement antibody into the experiments.

The time cultures are allowed to grow certainly is of major
importance and it might be possible that some stimulation is
missed if cultures are terminated after 5 instead of 6 or 7 days.

In addition to technical drawbacks which arise mostly in isolating tumor cells the need for a great number of cultures to
control for unspecific stimulants makes the MLTC a very complicated method. In our hands it is almost never possible to
include all the necessary controls mentioned above, a difficulty
which could be overcome by a micro culture method.

The extent of stimulation in our laboratory never reaches that
of MLC or antigen-stimulated lymphocytes. This mild stimulation has been described and extensively discussed by other
authors too (7, 8, 9, 11). The weak mitogenicity of tumor cells

makes the evaluation of the results difficult. How this evaluation is done best is a controversial question. It is not easy to establish a net blastogenic index for the MLTC and probably each laboratory has to figure out itself what is to be considered significant stimulation in their hands. For exact statistical interpretation more complicated tests with analysis of variance have to be done. Furthermore no increase in DNA-synthesis in the MLTC test when compared to the controls does not exclude host-tumor immune reactions. It could indicate,for instance,that there are no antigens on the respective tumor cells, that the antigens on the tumor cell have been coated in vivo by antibodies, that the lymphocyte receptors were blocked by surplus antigen shed by the tumor in vivo or on the basis of some other mechanism are not able to recognize tumor-specific antigens in vitro, that lymphocytes reactive to tumor cells are trapped in the lymph node stations draining the tumor site and cannot be isolated from peripheral blood, etc. The MLTC test in this respect needs further critical evaluation.

Although it was not the aim of this contribution to present results or to discuss the specificity and sensitivity of the MLTC for the demonstration of host-tumor immune reactions some results are given in conclusion. We find positive autologous cultures in 5-20% of tumor patients and up to 50% in the homologous situation. Correlation to skin tests and other in vitro assays is bad, probably because each system measures different immunological events. Although a disease-related behaviour of lymphocyte transformation in vitro has been observed (15, 16) until now no general statement is possible as to whether a positive MLTC has any prognostic value.

Summary

The mixed lymphocyte tumor cell culture as a laboratory method to demonstrate tumor-specific immunity is extensively described. Technical problems of the method are discussed.

References

1. LING, N.R. (1968), Lymphocyte Stimulation, North-Holland Publ. Amsterdam, J. Wiley & Sons Inc., New York.

2. BAIN, B., VAS, M.R. & LOWENSTEIN, L. (1964), Blood 23, 108.

3. BACH, F.H., BOCK, H., GRAUPNER, K., DAY, E. & KLOSTERMANN, H. (1969), Proc. Nat. Acad. Sci. 62, 377.

4. PIESSENS, W.F., WYBRAN, J., MANASTER, J. & STRIJCKMANS, P.A. (1970), Blood 36, 421.

5. SAVEL, H. (1969), Cancer 24, 56.

6. JEHN, U.W., NATHANSON, L., SCHWARTZ, R.S. & SKINNER, M. (1970), N. Engl. J. Med. 283, 329.

7. STJERNSWÄRD, J., CLIFFORD, P., SINGH, S. & SVEDMYR, E. (1968), E. Afr. Med. J. 45, 484.

8. NAGEL, G.A., STARNEAULT, G., HOLLAND, J.F., KIRKPATRICK, D. & KIRKPATRICK, R. (1970), Cancer Res. 30, 1828.

9. VANKY, F., STJERNSWÄRD, J., KLEIN, G. & NILSONNE, U. (1971), J. Nat. Cancer Inst. 47, 95.

10. GUTTERMAN, J.U., ROSSEN, R.D., BUTLER, W.T., McCREDIE, K.B., BODEY, G.P., FREIREICH, R.J. & HERSH, E.M. (1973), N. Engl. J. Med. 288, 169.

11. MAVLIGIT, G.M., GUTTERMAN, J.U., McBRIDE, C.M. & HERSH, E.M. (1973) Nat. Cancer Inst. Monogr. 37, 167.

12. BÖYUM, A. (1968), Scand. J. Clin. Lab. Invest. 21, Suppl. 97, 77.

13. PPO = 2.5-diphenyloxazol ($C_{15}H_{11}NO$)
POPOP = 2.2'-p-phenylen-bis (4-methyl-5-phenyloxazol) ($C_{26}H_{20}N_2O_2$)

14. HAN, T., MOORE, G.E. & SOKAL, J.E. (1971), Proc. Soc. Exp. Biol. Med. 136, 976.

15. VIZA, D.C., BERNARD-DEGANI, O., BERNARD, C. & HARRIS, R. (1969), Lancet II, 493.

16. NAGEL, G.A., PIESSENS, W.F., STILMANT, M.M. & LEJEUNE, F. (1971), Eur. J. Cancer 7, 41.

1.4 Lymphocyte Tansformation in Malignant Diseases. Communication I: Methodologic Problems

A. Pappas and P. G. Scheurlen

Already in the beginning ot the 20th century MAXIMOW drew attention to the pluripotency of lymphocytes (1). However it was only in the course of the modern development taken by immunology and immunegenetics that the special role was recognized these cells play in immune processes and that it was found that lymphocytes are the carriers of cellular immune reaction and particularly the small thymus-dependent lymphocytes, the so-called T-lymphocytes, that can be shown in the blood (2). NOWELL made an essential contribution to this when in 1960 he observed that phytohaemagglutinin in addition to its well-known erythro- and leuco-agglutinating capacities is able to activate blood-lymphocytes to transformation in culture (3). This phenomenon is closely related to the morphological and biological changes of lymphocytes during immunological reaction in vivo. The lymphocyte transformation test under the influence of phytohaemagglutinin (PHA) has made an important contribution in the field of immunology and cell-biology and in particular for testing the capacity of the cellular immune system to react in various diseases. (4, 5, 6, 7, 8, 9, 10).

Our experience with the lymphocyte transformation test is based on 200 cultures from healthy test persons and 150 cultures from patients suffering from reticular and lympho-proliferative diseases as well as from carcinoma patients (see part II). The age of the control persons was between 20 and 50 years, with an average of 30 years.

Methods

1. Preparation of the cell suspension

20-40 ml venal blood is drawn up in 20 ml plastic syringes with an added 1000 IU Heparin (Liquemin)^R for each one. After spontaneous sedimentation for 2-3 hours at 37°C in the syringe in an upright position the supernatant plasma, rich in cells, is transferred into a sterile container with a curved cannula. The suspension is mixed by slight shaking, then the leucocytes are counted in a NEUBAUER counting chamber and the relative number of lymphocytes determined by means of a differential smear. This gives the absolute lymphocyte content of the suspension. By dilution or concentration of the cell suspension with autologous plasma the number of lymphocytes is stabilized at 2000 lymphocytes/ mm^3. In order to avoid damage to the cells the substance is centrifuged for 10 min. at 150 x g (900 rpm with a radius of 16 cm). When special questions are to be answered, for example for testing the effect of the granulocytes in the culture we separate the lymphocytes out of the other cells by means of a RABINOWITZ column with nylon fibres (Leuco Pak 4 C 2401 Fenwal Laboratories, Illinois) and glass beads. For this purpose the suspension rich in leucocytes is diluted 1:2 with HANK's solution previously warmed to 37°C and poured into the previously rinsed column already warmed to 37°C. The glass column is 40 cm long and has an interior diameter of 2.5 cm. It is brought to 37° by means of a cooling shell. The filling of the column is done in stages of 4 cm nylon cotton wool for each one. After every one of the stages a 4 cm thick layer of siliconized glass beads is inserted. The column which had already been sterilized in an

autoclave is pre-rinsed with cell-free plasma. Next the leuco-
cyte-rich plasma is added in such a way that it completely pene-
trates the nylon cotton wool respectively the glass bead zones.
The column remains closed for 30 min. and only then the cells
are received in a sterile tube. The degree of purity of the so
separated lymphocyte suspensions lies by 90 - 95%. For examinations of the metabolism on lymphocytes, thrombocytes and
erythrocytes were removed by means of further processing of
the cell suspension: the plasma containing lymphocytes is
mixed with the double quantity of aqua bidest. and after careful
decanting is centrifuged off during 5 min. at low speed (150 x g).
The supernatant is rejected and the lymphocyte sediment resuspended in medium TL 199 (Difco) or in autologous heparin
plasma. The degree of purity of the so separated lymphocyte
suspension in our tests lay between 90 and 95 %.

2. Preparation of culture

The samples for culture are placed into Packard screw-up
tubes with a liquid content of 20 ml. Medium TL 199 was used.
It has to be pre-heated to 37° in the incubator before preparation. The culture dishes contain 2 ml cell suspension and 8 ml
medium as well as the pertinent stimulant, as mentioned above.
The cell number is stabilised to 2000 lymphocytes/mm^3. The
dose for PHA (Difco) is of 0.1 ml per 10 ml liquid culture. All
tests are made on 3 samples. Every time the optimal dosage for
the strongest lymphocyte transformation was determined with
different PHA concentrations. The following preparations were
tested: a) PHA Difco P, b) unpurified and c) purified PHA
Wellcome. The PHA preparations are always added in a concentration of 0.0025, 0.005, 0.01, 0.02, 0.03, 0.04, 0.05 and
0.06 ml per ml culture.

After determining the optimal stimulating dose (see Fig. 1) all
tests were exclusively made with the concentration determined
by the test (0.01 ml PHA-P Difco per ml prepared culture).

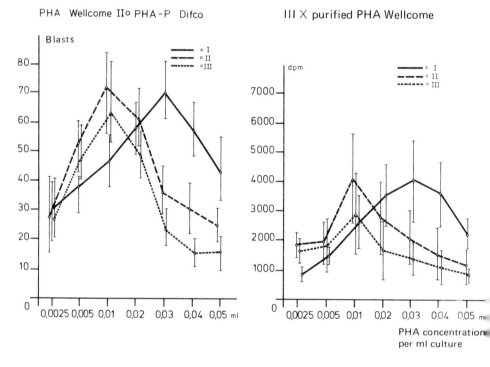

Fig.1. Dependency of transformation rate [blast %] and of 14 C
thymidine-incorporation [dpm] of the PHA concentration in the
culture.

After sterile covering with aluminium foil and screwing up the
containers with a lid the cultures are placed in the incubator
where they are kept at $37^{\circ}C$. The duration of the incubation
varies with the objective of the test. After sterile preparation
the cultures may be kept up to 11 days, however after the 5th
respectively 7th day the vessels containing the culture must be

aired and the pH value brought to 7.4 without change of medium. Cultures from patients with lympho- and reticuloproliferative diseases were observed up to 11 days in accordance with the object.

3. Taking up of the cultivated cells and evaluation of the preparations with light-microscope

After the end of incubation the sediment is carefully removed with a teflon-coated glass-rod. Once the cell-suspension has been transferred into a centrifuge tube and has been centrifuged (150 x g) the supernatant is drawn off with a pipette and rejected; small drops of the concentrated cell-sediment are then smeared onto a slide. After drying in air and fixation of the preparations with glacial acetic acid alcohol (3 parts absolute alcohol and 1 part glacial acetic acid) at $4^{O}C$ for 30 min. the smears were stained following PAPPENHEIM.

For judging the transformation rate by means of light-microscope 1000 cells with round nuclei are differentiated out, a distinction is made between lymphocytes, transitional forms, blasts, so-called PHA cells and macrophages. Special attention was given to the presence of mitoses.

4. Determination of the ^{14}C thymidine-incorporation of the cultivated cells by means of the fluid scintillation measurement.

Due to the leucoagglutinating property of the PHA it is frequently difficult, even impossible, to arrive at an exact morphological evaluation of the transformation. With the fluid scintillation spectrometry we now have a method which permits of reliable quantitative determinations. ^{14}C and ^{3}H thymidine as soft beta-radiators are directly added to the fluid scintillators, this makes it possible to keep the measuring arrangement simple.

Counting gives the average incorporation value of the total cell-population, whereby one obtains a cross-section of the proliferation activity of a determined number of cells in the culture.

90 minutes before the end of cultivation time samples are carefully swung backwards and forwards and one half (5 ml) of the culture transferred into a sterile container. 0.5 ml ^{14}C thymidine with an activity of 0.5 μC is added to the remaining portion (thymidine-2-C-14, Fa.NEN, specific activity 56 m C/mM dissolved in medium TC 199). The labeled as well as the unlabeled portion of the culture samples are then submitted to further incubation at 37°C for 90 min. After that light-microscopic preparations are made of the unlabeled half of the culture. The growth of the cells of the sample to which ^{14}C thymidine had been added is stopped by dipping into icewater and by adding 5 ml of cold medium TC 199. Ten minutes later the culture is centrifuged at 4°C and 400 x g during 10 min. The supernatant is pipetted off down to 1 ml and the cell sediment is stirred up. After a dropwise addition of 1 ml 20% trichloro-acetic-acid (TCA) and another centrifugation at 4° C and 1100 x g during 10 min. the supernatant is removed down to 0.5 ml and the sediment washed out in 5 ml 5% TCA solution. The total content of the sample is filtered through a Sartorius membrane filter (pore size 0.2 μ size 25 mm SM 11307) so that the cells will adhere to the filter layer. After rinsing twice with 10 ml 5 % TCA the filter is carefully lifted from the frit with a pair of forceps (SM 16624) and with the cell layer upward is placed on a filter-paper where it is dried at 80°C for 24 hours, dissolved in sheets of low-pressure-polyethylene of NEN Chemical GmbH in 10 ml Aquasol (NEN) and measured twice during 20 min. in fluid scintillation counter (Intertechnique). The impulse values are corrected to

zero-effect and fluorescence-solution and recorded in degrada-
tions per minute (dpm).

5. Autoradiography: In vitro determination of the generation
   cycle and its part phases of the blood lymphocytes stimulated with PHA.

The proliferation kinetics of phytohaemagglutinin-stimulated
peripheral lymphocytes was determined autoradiographically
with the help of the ^{3}H and ^{14}C thymidine double-labeling system
according to HILSCHER and MAURER (11), WIMBER and
QUASTLER 12 and of the "%-labeled mitosis" method of
QUASTLER and SHERMAN (13).

a) ^{3}H labeling index

Observation time for cultures for this test amounts to 216 hours
9 culture samples are prepared out of every lymphocyte suspension, to one sample every 24 hours 10 μC thymidine-methyl-^{3}H
(NEN Chemicals GmbH, specific activity 2 mC/mM) in 1 ml
medium TC 199 is added. Next the sample is kept in the incubator at 37°C for 1 hour. In order to obtain cells for the smears
the suspension is transferred into a pointed centrifuge tube and
centrifuged for 10 min. at 150 x g. Supernatant medium is rejected and the cells left at the bottom of the little tube are drawn
up with a Pasteur pipette and smeared over the slides previously cleaned with methanol. After drying the smears are fixed for
three minutes in ethanol acetic acid (3:1) and afterwards washed
for one hour in a solution of aqua dest. and in active thymidine for
the removal of the non-incorporated thymidine-methyl ^{3}H. After
drying the smears the autoradiograph emulsion is laid on according to the DIP coating method. For pure ^{3}H labeled preparations the K^2 emulsion (ILFORD, London) is used. The
smears are dipped into the emulsion diluted 1:2 with aqua dest.

so that a thin film is spread over the smears like a photographic coating. Next the preparations are air-dried in an upright position, in complete darkness for 8 hours and for 11 days are exposed in sealed wrapping. After photographic development and fixation the autoradiograms are stained with hematoxin for easier evaluation of the nuclei, washed for one hour under flowing water from the main, rinsed in aqua destillata and finally imbedded in gelatine.

b) Mitosis index

Part of the smears prepared to determine the ^{3}H thymidine labelling index are stained following PAPPENHEIM and the number of mitoses determined for 1000 cells.

c) Double-labelling tests

Of every one of the lymphocyte suspensions to be examined 4 samples are prepared. After cultivation for 72, 96, 120 and 144 hours 1 sample is always incubated in the incubator with 1 μC thymidine-2 ^{14}C specific activity 25-30 mC/ml NEN Chemicals GmbH) in 1 ml medium TC 199 for one hour and after that washed twice with non-radio-active thymidine.For this purpose the suspension is transferred into a sterile flat-bottomed centrifuge glass, centrifuged at 600 x g for 30 sec and the supernatant medium drawn off with a sterile syringe. After adding an equal quantity of fresh medium with inactive thymidine the cells are evenly distributed by shaking the glass. Then centrifuging is repeated the medium removed and an equal quantity of fresh medium as well as 11 μC thymidine-methyl ^{3}H is added. After this the sample is placed in the incubator for another 60 minutes. The smears are made and fixed the same as the preparations labeled with ^{3}H. But unlike these they are coated with 65 emulsion (ILFORD, London). Afterwards they are airdried for 24 hours in complete darkness and then exposed for 8 days. With regard to fixation, staining and imbedding the double-label-ed autoradiograms are from thereon treated in the same way as the preparations labeled with ^{3}H.

d) <u>Determination of the first appearance of labeled mitoses</u>

For this examination three samples for culture are prepared from every lymphocyte suspension. After the cell culture has developed in the incubator for 96 hours every sample is given an injection of 10 μC thymidine-methyl ^{3}H. Every 2 hours after the ^{3}H thymidine application smears are made of one sample, - so that the last sample of which smears are made had been incu-bated with ^{3}H thymidine for 16 hours. After a 3 minute fixation of the preparations in ethanol acetic acid 3:4 and one hour further washing in aqua destillata with inactive thymidine the au-toradiograms are then made according to the method indicated above for ^{3}H labeled smears.

Proliferation kinetics were calculated with the following formulae:

1) $^3H - I = \dfrac{S}{T}$

2) $^3H - I_{theor.} = \dfrac{^3H - I_{exper.}}{GF}$

3) $T_c : \nu \cdot \Delta t \cdot \dfrac{\ln 2}{T} = 1 - \dfrac{1}{1 + {}^3H - I \cdot e^{-\frac{\ln 2\,(G2 + M)}{T}}}$

4) $T_s : S = \dfrac{T}{\ln 2} \cdot \ln \left(1 + {}^3H - I \cdot e^{-\frac{\ln 2\,(G2 + M)}{T}}\right)$

I	= Index	T_s	= DNA Synthesis Time
S	= DNA Synthesis Phase	e	= e-function
T	= Generation Time	G2	= Growth Phase 2 (pre-mitotic phase)
theor.	= theoretical	M	= Duration of Mitosis
exper.	= experimental	ν	= value of the relation of the frequency of ^{14}C-nuclei (with and without ^{3}H) to pure ^{3}H-labeled nuclei
GF	= Growth Fraction		
T_c	= Generation Time		
Δt	= interval between the application of ^{14}C- and ^{3}H-thymidine		

the so-called theoretic ^{3}H labeling index is calculated from
equation ^{3}H-I theor.= ^{3}H - I exp: GF following HEMPEL, where
GF = growth fraction (15).

Since the factually proliferating lymphocytes multiply in the
PHA culture the actual duration of generation (Tc) and the
duration of the DNA synthesis phase (Ts) had to be found according to the evaluation method of LENNARTZ et al. (16). For Tc
(formula no. 3) for Ts (formula no. 4) Tc can be solved graphi-
cally if both sides are at first considered separately as functions
of T. When Tc is known, Ts can be determined by calculation
(10).

6. Chromatographic characteristics of an inhibiting factor in
    the serum of patients with malignant tumors.

Lymphocyte transformation in vitro after stimulation with PHA
is significantly reduced in patients with lymphogranulomatosis
(stage III-IV) in cases of chronic lymphatic leucemia and in
malignant tumors (see 6.1, page 319) . In previous publications we
drew attention to the fact that inhibition of lymphocyte transformation in malignant diseases may have a plasma factor as a
contributing cause (17, 19).

The plasma of carcinoma patients and healthy controls was
separated by chromatography with sephadex G 200 (particle size
40 - 120 μ, Pharmacia Chine Chemicals, Uppsala, Sweden) in
0.1 mol Tris (pH 7.4). The chromatographic column was 100
cm long and had a diameter of 2.5 cm. Applying this method we
obtained 4 fractions from the plasma (peak I-IV) when fractions
I, II and III corresponded to the usual serum protein fractions.

By rechromatography of the IVth fraction over Sephadex G 25
superfine (particle size 10-14 μ, Pharmacia Uppsala, Sweden)

we obtained 3 further fractions (peak IVa, IVb and IVc). All fractions were subsequently reduced to the original concentration and immediately before being added to the lymphocyte cultures they were sterilized by means of a bacteria frit.

Cultures were prepared with lymphocytes from tuberculin-sensitive persons according to the method described above. PHA or purified tuberculin were used as stimulants (PPD). Autologous plasma was rejected, so that the tuberculin-sensitive lymphocytes from healthy persons were cultivated with patients' plasma, respectively with the fractions obtained by chromatography(2 ml).

7. "in vivo" lymphocyte culture in the diffusion chamber

Millipore filters no. VCWP 0 1300, pore size 0.1 μ are firmly glued onto a plexi glass ring (millipore No. PROO 01410, 14 mm outside $\emptyset$, 10 mm inside $\emptyset$, 2 mm strong) using MF cement (millipore-MF-cement no. XX 7000000) and the appropriate special instrument. The filling of the autoclaved diffusion chamber with pure lymphocyte suspension and PHA additive is carried out with a tuberculin syringe. The orifice is then sealed with 2-3 drops of MF cement. After anaesthesizing white rats - weighing 200-250 g - with Nembutal and after a sterile medial incision into the abdominal wall has been performed, 3-4 of the filled diffusion chambers are implanted in the peritoneal cavity. Tests are interrupted the next day by killing the animals, the diffusion chambers are removed, their content is transferred into centrifugal glasses and centrifuged for 10 minutes (150 x g), Smears are made from the sediment fixed with glacial acetic acid alcohol and stained according to PAPPENHEIM.

Out of every series of examinations prepared cultures are labeled with ^{3}H thymidine for autoradiographic DNA synthetis after removal from the peritoneal cavity. Two diffusion chambers are

placed into a sterile culture dish containing 1 ml ^{3}H thymidine
methyl. One hour later the material is processed as described
above and the smears coated with K2 emulsion. Time of exposi-
tion: 10 days.

Results:

1. Dependence of blast formation respectively C^{14} thymidin
   incorporation of PHA concentration in the culture.

Number of blasts and C^{14} thymidine incorporation of the cells in
the culture depend on the strength of the PHA concentration in
the culture (Fig. 1). For purified PHA Wellcome and PHA-P-
Difco the optimal concentration was about 0.01 ml per ml of
culture. For the total extract of the Wellcome firm the optimal
concentration was 0.3 ml. Higher concentrations have a cytotoxic effect while lower doses were possibly insufficient for the
activation of all competent cells.

2. Morphological criteria, transformation rates on C^{14} respectively H^3 thymidine incorporation of the blood lymphocytes stimulated by PHA.

72 hours after the start of incubation in the presence of PHA
one finds the "blastlike" cells having a large nucleus with
strongly basophilic cytoplasma. The chromatin of the nucleus
is loose and contains 1-2 nucleolii. We found two forms of blast-
like cells in the cultures of healthy persons, so-called PHA
cells [20] : a immune blastlike cells with numerous polyriboso-
mes and only few cellorganelles and b) cells rich in RNA
(ribosomes) and mitochondriae, containing only little ergasto-
plasma. A GOLGI-apparatus and/or a centrosoma were frequently observed. Some of these cells resembled lymphoblasts.

After 72 hours of incubation the number of cells transformed to
resemble blasts in the culture on average was around 71%

(Fig. 4). The C^{14} thymidine incorporation of cultivated lymphocytes reached its maximum after 72 respectively 96 hours after the start of stimulation (Fig. 2). It then dropped quickly to a plateau between the 144th and the 216th hour (300-600 dpm) (Fig. 2). Figure 3 shows the course of the ^{3}H labeling index and the mitosis rate dependent on the age of the lymphocyte culture over a period of 216 hours. In all cases examined the number of the cells labeled with ^{3}H thymidine increased continuously up to a peak at 72 respectively 96 hours after the start of incubation. In the 216 hours cultures it was possible to show the cells respectively mitosis which in the 24 hours cultures were only slightly marked. In the control tests - lymphocyte cultures without added PHA - we rarely found 0.5 to 1% blasts and only very little C^{14} thymidine incorporation (Fig. 2).

The reproducibility of the method was checked on 50 cultures from healthy persons (Fig. 4 and 5). Blood lymphocytes of healthy controls were stimulated with PHA twice in 5 days. The transformation rate, as well as the C^{14} thymidine incorporation showed no significant deviation (Fig. 4 and 5). The presence of granulocytes in the culture does not seem to influence the blast transformation noticeably, in tests with "pure" lymphocytes the transformation values were the same as in cultures prepared . with leucocytes (Fig. 6).

3. Cell kinetic data of lymphocytes stimulated with PHA
of healthy persons resulted on average as shown below:
a) DNA synthesis phase 14, 16 hours,
b) Minimum duration of the G-2-phase; 2 hours,
c) Factual generation time: 30.5 hours.

4. Lymphocyte transformation through PHA in the diffusion
   chamber (in vivo).

With this experimental procedure we found the highest values

for blast transformation and ^{3}H labeling index after 72 hours

with subsequent continuous drop until the 264th hour (Fig. 7).

In the control test we found no signs of a transformation and only

now and then a negligeable ^{3}H thymidine incorporation.

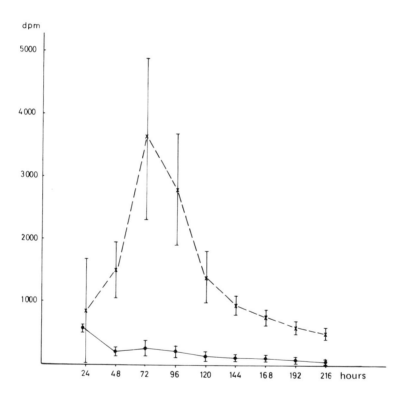

Fig. 2. ^{14}C thymidine incorporation in PHA stimulated lymphocytes of healthy donors as a function of the duration of incubation
(broken line). Control test (full line). The activity measured
was indicated in dpm.

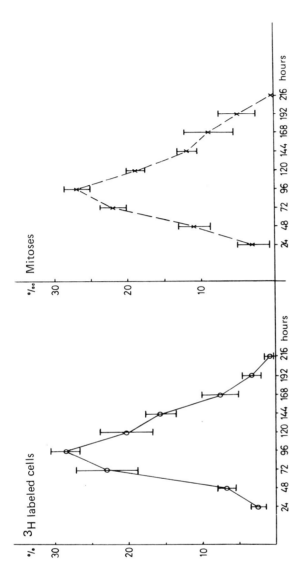

Fig. 3. ^{3}H labeling index and index of mitosis of the PHA stimulated lymphocytes of healthy persons as a function of the duration of incubation.

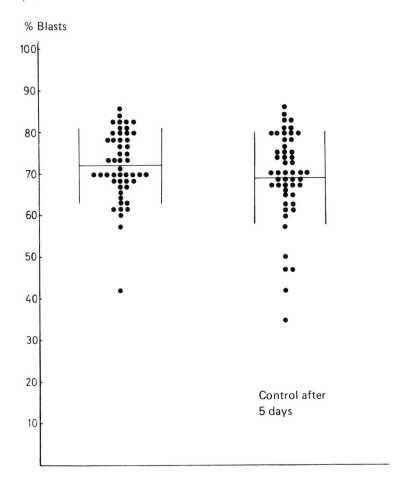

Fig. 4. Transformation rate after two bloodwithdrawals (in 5 days) taken from healthy test persons.

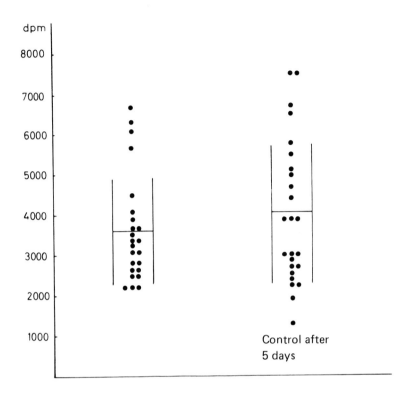

Fig. 5. ^{14}C thymidine incorporation of the PHA stimulated lymphocytes of healthy test persons after two blood withdrawals in 5 days.

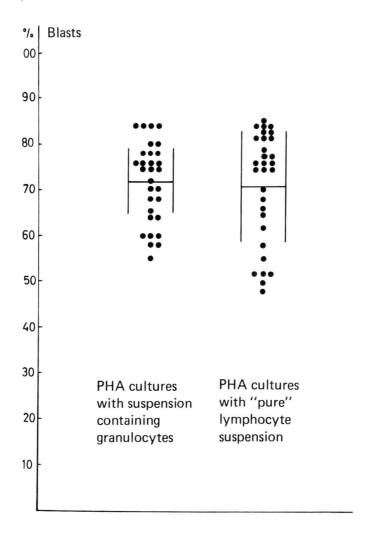

Fig. 6. Granulocytes respectively monocytes do not influence the PHA transformation of normal lymphocytes. 30 PHA cultures of healthy persons were simultaneously prepared separately with leucocyte and "pure" lymphocyte suspensions. In each case the portion of blasts without mitoses found in the 3 days cultures was indicated.

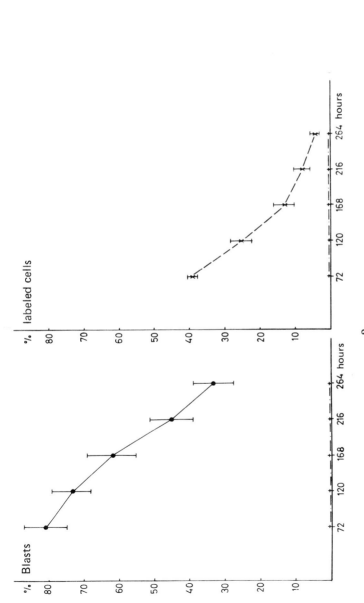

Fig. 7. Transformation (blast %) and ^{3}H index of the PHA stimulated lymphocytes of healthy controls in a diffusion chamber ("in vivo")

Discussion

A large part of the progress achieved in recent years in the
field of cellular immunity is doubtless due to the development of
in vitro systems for tissue culture. By isolating and cultivating
certain types of cells it became possible to explain biochemical
processes such as proliferation, RNA and DNA synthesis and antibody production independent of other cell populations. Lymphocyte transformation in vitro under the influence of unspecific mi-
togenes (PHA, Pokeweed-mitogen, Concanavalin A and others)
or after stimulation with specific antigens in recent years was
used by numerous research workers to explore and interpret
cellular immunity (survey in 10 and 21). The lymphocyte transformation test proved to be a practicable method also in the
clinic insofar as for a series of diseases one can prove clear
parallels between a cellular immune defect in vivo and the in
vitro transformation capacity of the blood lymphocytes (see
6.1, page 326).

Though morphological criteria for blast formation have been
laid down, interpretation of the results obtained by different
working groups is made difficult through differences in methodology. Widely varying opinions are held on type and dose of anti-
coagulants used (22). According to our experience 50 U Heparin
per ml blood proved to be optimal. Other authors observed no
effect on the lymphocyte metabolism with doses up to 500 U/ml
while WINKLER found an inhibition of the aminoacid incorporation in lymphocytes already from 50-100 U/ml (22). An accelera-
tion of the erythrocyte sedimentation through macromolecular
substances (23) was not indispensible in our experimental procedure. Some authors report on unfavourable experience with
dextran in mouse-blood, while others were able to achieve better

sedimentation of the erythrocytes by using high molecular dex-
trans also in the blood of mice and guinea pigs.

Our findings which agree with the results obtained by other
working groups (25) are that the presence of granulocytes and
monocytes in the culture do not influence PHA transformation
of the lymphocytes. No significant differences were found in the
formation of blasts and in the ^{14}C thymidine incorporation when
"pure" lymphocytes or lymphocyte cultures with granulocytes
were prepared in which PHA was present. However, the transformation rate after stimulation with specific antigens in pure
lymphocyte cultures was reduced by comparison with cultures
containing monocytes as well as granulocytes (25, 26, 27).

TÄRNVIK found an increased ^{3}H thymidine incorporation of the
lymphocytes incubated with PHA when these had been cultivated
with leucocytes and erythrocytes present. It is also held that
erythrocytes and erythrocyte membranes added to the PHA
culture can increase the DNA synthesis of the lymphocytes
(28, 29).

A PHA concentration (PHA-P-Difco and purified PHA Wellcome)
of 0.01 ml per culture prepared and 4×10^{6} lymphocyte culture
proved to be optimal in our tests. Other authors recorded the
strongest lymphocyte transformation respectively C^{14} thymidine
incorporation with a markedly lower PHA dose (30, 31). It must
however be taken into consideration that our methodology devi-
ates considerably from the examination procedures described.
Because of the strict sterile conditions of work on our laboratory
we have dispensed with adding antibiotics. We also quite inten-
tionally did not cultivate with calf-serum present in order not to
influence the possible effect of a plasma factor in cases of
carcinoma (see page 68).

It is frequently difficult to achieve a precise morphological evaluation of blast-transformation by counting the blast ratio in the
culture. The reason being the well-known agglutinating property of
PHA which often does not permit of a reliable classification of
individual cells. Some authors dissolve the agglutinates by means
of a hypotonic sodium citrate solution and mild fixation (32);
subsequently the nuclei are stained with orcein and classified
according to size and structure. We were able to achieve good
conditions for differentation when by means of a PASTEUR-pipette
little drops from the concentrated cellular sediment were plated
out carefully and evenly.

Determination of the cell content at the time of measurement
constitutes a further parameter for judging lymphocyte transformation. Precise cell counts in the counting chamber or with
the Coulter counter cannot be carried out accurately as long as
agglutination persists. Two procedures for better countability
can be carried out relatively simply: Demonstration of the
nuclei after treatment with Pronase (SERVA, Heidelberg) or by
dissolving the agglutinates through treatment with 0.1 ml
Cetavlon cetrimide B.P. 40% w/vI.C.E. and subsequent
counting of the whole cells.

Isotope-incorporation into the cells forms an objective and
reproducible method for judging lymphocyte transformation
under the influence of PHA as well as under that of specific antigens. This does not only allow to detect the percentage of labeled cells, but also to estimate that of the granules, the DNA
synthesis inside individual cells. While our autoradiographic
results tally with the findings of other workers (34, 35, 36) the
C^{14} thymidine incorporation values measured by fluid scintillation
spectrometry frequently cannot be compared with the results

obtained by other authors. This is obviously due to the difference in measuring techniques applied. MICHALOWSKI (37) carried out measurements of activity with the gas flow counting tube. Here only part of the substance to be measured is considered since only a diluted aliquote part is pipetted into the measuring vessel and evaporated to a film. There exists an interdependence between measuring yield and film. On the other hand fluid scintillation spectrometry offers a series of advantages: The cells are cultivated and stimulated in the counting vessel itself, so that losses through pipetting can be avoided. Another advantage lies in measuring the whole culture. This method was modified by AISENBERG (38) so that the entire culture was filtered after TCA precipitation. We adopted this procedure for our own tests in a slightly modified form. The labeled cell sediment remains on the surface of the filter while the culture liquid can be removed without loss of material. Consequently our measured values are much lower than comparable ones of other authors. We found a far-reaching parallelism between rate of transformation and measured C^{14} thymidine incorporation. This is in accordance with the findings of other working groups.

Kinetic findings of proliferation of PHA stimulated lymphocytes from healthy persons are rarely reported in literature. COOPER and co-workers (40) as well as QUAGLINO and HAYHOE (41) in their cultures found a minimum duration of the G 2-phase of 2-3 hours, - a value we were able to confirm in our tests. Further the DNA synthesis phase was of 14 hours and actual generation time 30 1/2 hours. No greater fluctuations occurred between the various cultures prepared.

C^{14} thymidine incorporation of the normal lymphocytes cultivated with PHA or PPD with the serum fractions present which had been separated by chromatography over sephadex G 200 - if the serum came from healthy donors - lay within the standard area. Neither did the low molecular fraction, possibly a peptide or a nucleoproteid influence blast formation (see 6.1, page 324).

The diffusion chamber method "in vivo" introduced by ALGIRE et al (40) in our view is the preferred method for longtime obser-vation of stimulated lymphocytes. In this experimental procedure the body fluid is diffused through the filter membranes and con-stitutes and optimal culture medium. In this way damaging pH deviation and temperature fluctuation as well as the development of toxic substances can be avoided.

A change of medium in longtime cultures in vitro can considerab-ly affect transformation (41). In lymphocytes incubated in vitro with specific antigens this effect is probably due to soluble factors formed by the sensitized lymphocytes (44,45). With a daily change of medium thymidine incorporation of activated lymphocytes is doubled in the PHA culture.

The possibility to watch cultures over a longer period without medium by means of the diffusion chamber method is another advantage of this experimental procedure. It must however be said that this is a heterologous system and that large molecules can easily pass the membrane, a fact which could lead to meta-bolic exchange processes between the incubated cells and the host animal, thus making test conditions more complex than in the culture (42).

The lymphocyte transformation test in vitro doubtless consti-tutes a method of importance for research into the cellular im-mune phenomena. Well arranged experimental procedures permit of answers to clinical questions. The divergent results obtained by some scientists in this field in our opinion show up the necessity to standardize methodology in order to be able to use the lymphocyte transformation test for clinical diagnostics.

Experimental work was supported by a grant from the Deutsche Forschungsgemeinschaft (pa 129) .

References

1. MAXIMOW, A. A. [1909], Folia Haematol. , Frankfurt, 8 , 125

2. FUDENBERG, H. H. , GOOD, R. A. , HITZIG, W. , KUNKEL, H. G. , ROITT, I. M. , ROSEN, F. S. , ROWE, D. S. , SELIGMANN, M. & SOOTHILL, J. R. [1970], N. Engl. J. Med. 283, 656

3. NOWELL, P.C. [1960], Cancer Res. 20, 462

4. COOPER, H. L. & RUBIN, A. D. [1966], Science 152, 516

5. RUBIN, A. D. [1970], Blood 35, 708

6. HIRSCHHORN, R. , BRITTINGER, G. , HIRSCHHORN, K. & WEISSMANN, G. [1968], J. Cell. Biol. 37, 412

7. HALPERN, B. & ROBINEAUX, R. [1968], Bull. Soc. Clin. Biol. 5-6, 4059

8. PERLMAN, P. & HOLM, G. [1969], Adv. Immunology 11, 117

9. LAWRENCE, H. S. & LANDY, M. [1969], Mediators of Cellular Immunity, Acad. Press, New York

10. PAPPAS, A. [1971], Die Lymphozytenkultur: Methodik und klinische Anwendung, Habilitationsschrift

11. HILSCHER, W. & MAURER, W. [1962], Naturwissenschaften 49, 352

12. PILGRIM, Ch. & MAURER, W. [1962], Naturwissenschaften 49, 544

13. WIMBER, D. E. & QUASTLER, H. [1963], Exp. Cell. Res. 30, 8

14. HEMPEL, K. [1968], Virchow Arch. B. Zellpathol. 1, 15

15. MENDELSON, M. L. [1962], J. Nat. Cancer Inst. 28, 1015

16. LENNARTZ, K.-J. , MAURER, W. & EDER, M. [1968], Histochemie 13, 84

17. PAPPAS,A. & SCHEURLEN,P.G.[1968],Verh.Deut.Ges. Inn.Med. 74, 1254

18. SCHEURLEN,P.G.,SCHNEIDER,W.& PAPPAS,A.[1971], Lancet II, 1265

19. SCHEURLEN,P.G. & PAPPAS,A.[1971],Verh.Deut.Ges. Inn.Med. 77, 749

20. ORFANOS,C.,PAPPAS,A.& SCHEURLEN,P.G.[1969], Z.Gesamte Exp.Med. 149, 283

21. HUBER,H.,PASTNER,D.& GABL,F.[1972],Laboratori- umsdiagnose hämatologischer und immunologischer Erkran- kungen,Springer-Verlag, Berlin

22. HAVEMANN,K.[1971], in Leukozytenkulturen. Verhandlungs- bericht der 2.Arbeitstagung über Leukozytenkulturen [eds. Brittinger,G. und Roggenbach,H.J.], F.K.Schattauer-Ver- lag, Stuttgart - New York

23. ANDERS,J.M.,MOORE,E.C. & EMANUEL,R.[1963], J.Med.Genet. 2, 57

24. COULSON,A.S. & CHALMERS,D.G.[1964],Lancet I, 468

25. HERSH,E.M. & HARRIS,I.E.[1968],J.Immunol. 100,1148

26. HUBER,H.,PASTNER,D.,SCHMALZE,F. & BRAUNSTEI- NER,H. [1969], Verh.Deut.Ges.Inn.Med. 35, 497

27. SEEGER,R.C. & OPPENHEIM,T.T.[1970],J.Exp.Med. 132, 44

28. TÄRNVIK,A.[1970],Acta Pathol.Microbiol.Scand.B 78,733

29. JOHNSON,R.A. & KIRKPATRICK,C.[1970],Fed.Proc.29,370

30. SCHELLEKENS,P.Th.A.[1970], a]Lymphocyte Transforma- tion in vitro,Thesis,Universiteit van Amsterdam,Drukkerig, "Aemstelstad" -Amsterdam - b] - & EIJSVOOGEL,V.P. [1968], Clin.Exp.Immunol. 3, 571

31. JUNGE,U.,HOEKSTRA,I.,WOLFE,L.& DEINHARDT,F. [1970], Clin.Exp.Immunol. 7, 431

32. HIRSCHHORN,K.[1968], in Human Transplantations [eds. Rapaport,F.T. and Dausset,T.], p.406, Grune Stratton- Publ. New York

33. STEWART,C.C.& INGRAM,M. [1967], Blood 29, 628

34. MacKINNEY,A.A.,STOHLMAN,F. & BRECHER,G.[1962], Blood, 19, 349

35. EPSTEIN, L. B. & STOHLMAN, F. jr. [1964], Blood 24, 69

36. YOFFEY, J. M., WINTER, G. C. B., OSMOND, D. G. & MEEK, E. S. [1965], Brit. J. Haematol. 11, 448

37. MICHALOWSKI, A. [1963], Exp. Cell Res. 32, 609

38. AISENBERG, A. C. [1965], Nature [London] 205, 1233

39. CARON, G. A., SARKANY, I., WILLIAMS, H. S., TODD, A. P. & GELL, H. M. C. [1965], Lancet II, 1266

40. ALGIRE, G. H., WEAVER, T. M. & PREHN, R. T. [1954], J. Nat. Cancer Inst. 15, 493

41. NILSSON, B. S. [1972], Cell Immunol. 3, 333

42. SCHUMACHER, K. [1971], in Leukozytenkulturen [eds. Brittinger, G. and Roggenbach, H. J.], F. K. Schattauer-Verlag, Stuttgart - New York

43. ORFANOS, C., PAPPAS, A., BERTRAM, R. & SCHEURLEN, P. G. [1970], Der Lymphozytentransformationstest [LTT] als Allergietest in vitro, in Allergie- und Immunitätsforschung [eds. Letterer, E. und Gronemeyer, W.], F. K. Schattauer-Verlag, Stuttgart - New York

44. KASAKURA, S. [1970], J. Immunol. 105, 1162

45. VALENTINE, F. T. & LAWRENCE, H. S. [1969], Science 165, 1014

1.5 Microcytotocicity Test for Detection of Cellular Immunity to Nephroblastoma in Man

V. Diehl

Accumulating data suggest tumor-related immunological reactions in man. In vitro studies have shown that tumor cells might differ antigenetically from normal cells. This is reflected by humoral and cell-mediated immune responses, directed against tumor specific surface antigens. Main emphasis has been put on the studies of the cell-mediated reactions, since, according to BURNET [1],this might reflect the main vector of immunological surveillance.

Some clinical observations in patients with nephroblastoma suggest possible immunological defence mechanisms. The prognosis is much poorer for cases with invasion of the regional lymphnodes than with invasion of the local blood vessels. Furthermore HELLSTRÖM [2] and coworkers have described cellular immunity in 2 out of 3 patients with nephroblastoma tested by the colony inhibition test.

In our investigation [DIEHL et al.[3]], JEREB et al.[4]] we used the microtechnique described by TAGASUKI and KLEIN to investigate the cell-mediated immunity in nephroblastoma patients against explanted autochthonus and allogeneic tumorcells.

Two different studies are described: firstly a vertical survey-study of 24 nephroblastoma patients in different stages of disease compared with the reactions of 24 control persons, and secondly a horizontal followup study of 10 patients tested subsequently during course of disease and treatment.

The techniques applied were briefly as follows:

Target cells: Tumor and normal cells from primary kidney tumors and lungmetastases were dispersed, trypsinized and used for testing either as primary or tissue passage cells.

Effector cells: 10-60 ml of peripheral blood were sedimented in a plastic syringe and the lymphocytes seperated from granulocytes by iron powder or nylon column seperation.

Cytotoxicity test: 100-200 trypsinized cells were suspended in 10 μl of medium and explanted in the 60 holes of the falcon plastic-test-plate, 12-24 hrs. prior to the addition of lymphocytes. Approximately 250-500 lymphocytes target cells were overlayed on the nearly confluent target cells layer. For all tests 2 control systems were used: a horizontal control in form of lymphocytes from control persons and a vertical in form of normal cells as target tissue. The test plates were incubated for 3-6 days in 37° [ca. 5% CO_2-air-atmosphere] incubators before the plates were then washed, fixed and stained for further evaluation. The number of surviving cells was counted and the results evaluated as seen Table 1.

The specific cytotoxicity was expressed in percentage cytotoxic reduction of explanted cells and calculated as the reaction of lymphocytes in relation to control lymphocytes, the non-specificity as the reaction of control lymphocytes in relation to number of surviving target cells incubated without lymphocytes [Tab. 1]. A test was considered as positive when the cytotoxicity of test lymphocytes exceeded that for control lymphocytes significantly and was greater on tumor than on normal tissue.

Table 1

Calculation of cytotoxic reactions

Percentage
specific
cytotoxicity

$$= \frac{\text{Surviving tumor cells treated with test lymphocytes}}{\text{Surviving tumor cells treated with control lymphocytes}} \times 100$$

Percentage
non-specific
cytotoxicity

$$= \frac{\text{Surviving tumor cells treated with control lymphocytes}}{\text{Surviving tumor cells with BME medium alone}} \times 100$$

Patients studied: In the first study 19 patients were tested against autochthonous and allogeneic tumor cells in vitro. At time of testing 8 patients had metastatic tumors, 11 were free of metastasis.

The control group consisted of healthy persons, patients with non malignant diseases and patients with tumors other than nephroblastoma.

The correlation between clinical stage and lymphocyte reactivity was examined [Tab. 2]. 2 out of 8 patients with disseminated disease [25%] had a stronger reaction on tumor tissue than control persons. Five out of 11 patients [45,5%] without dissemination, however, showed a higher cytotoxicity than control individuals.

This finding prompted further horizontal studies on 10 nephroblastoma patients during different phases of disease and treatment. Eight patients had disseminated disease, 2 were free of secondaries. The control group consisted of 22 age matched non-nephroblastoma children. All patients were tested between 3 and 5 times.

High cytotoxic in vitro reactivity was correlated to remission-phases [Fig. 1], and decreased during progress of disease. Therapy, depressing the total white blood cell count did not effect the specific cytotoxicity, since a low mononuclear count occured to the same degree in positive and negative reactors, with meanvalues of mononuclear cells of $1400/\text{mm}^3$.

The results summarized in the next table [Tab. 3] confirm the earlier described observation, that specific cytotoxicity is correlated to remission. Eleven out of 18 tests were positive [61%] when patients were free of tumors, as compared to only 1 positive test out of 15 [7%] during time of active disease.

Table 2

Cytotoxicity on tumor target tissue of lymphocytes from patients with nephroblastoma in relation to their clinical stages

	Micro-plate test		Total		
	tested	positive[1]	tested	positive	%positive
Patients with metastasis	8[3]	2	8	2	25
Patients without metastasis	11	5	11	5	45,5
Total	19	7	19	7	37

[1]Positive = significant at the 95-99.9% level.

[3]Number of patients

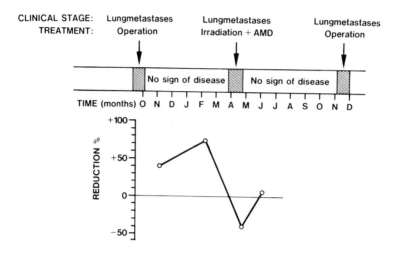

Fig. 1

Table 3

Cytotoxic reaction in relation to the phase of
nephroblastoma and treatment

		Cytotoxic tests		
		Positive	Total	Per cent positive
Active disease	Treatment	1	12	8
	No treatment	0	3	–
	Total	1	15	7
Disease in remission	Treatment	5	6	83
	No treatment	6	12	50
	Total	11	18	61

The results of this in vitro studies confirm the existance of tumor-related cellular immunity to nephroblastoma tumor cells. The specificity of these reactions is shown by the much lower reactivity of lymphocytes from patients with other tumors than nephroblastoma and the different reactivity of normal tissue tested in parallel to the tumor cells.

Variations in cytotoxic activity of the patients lymphocytes seem to be related to dissimination of disease. General lymphopenia does not parallel a decreased cytotoxic activity. The presented findings might reflect a true variation in tumor-related cytotoxicity with clinical status, but also might be due to a general decrease in immunologic reactivity.

Blocking antibodies, inhibiting lymphocyte reactivity in vivo, might account for the discrepancy between tumorprogress in vivo inspite of cytotoxic reactions against tumor cells in vitro.

References

1. BURNET, M.F. [1969], Cellular Immunity, Melbourne University Press, Cambridge University Press
2. HELLSTRÖM, I. , HELLSTRÖM , K.E., PIERCE, G.E. & YANG, J.P.S.[1968], Nature [London] 220, 1352
3. DIEHL, V. , JEREB, B. , STJERNSERÄRD, J. ,O TOOLE, C. & AHSTROEM, L.[1971], Int. J. Cancer 7, 277
4. JEREB, B. , DIEHL, V. & JUHLIN, J. , Relation between cellular immunity to nephroblastoma and the phase of the disease, Acta Paedriat. Scand. [in press].

1.6 Comparative Tumorimmunological Studies with the Microcytotoxicity Test and the DNA-Synthesis Inhibition Test

H. Warnatz

Several methods have been developed for the demonstration of immune mechanisms involved in the destruction of tumor target cells. Important factors which have to be taken in mind during selection of a convenient test system are

a] the properties of the tumor cells [growth characteristics, lysability of the tumor target cells],

b] the effector cells [amount and origin of the lymphocytes],

c] serum factors [antiserum, serum containing immune complexes].

In the present study we used the microcytotoxicity test and the DNA-synthesis inhibition test in order to examine whether they are capable to demonstrate cell-mediated immune reactions to tumor target cells and the interference of serum factors with the cellular immunity to tumor target cells. SV40 transformed fibroblasts from Balb/c mice [SV40TF] were used for immunization of isogeneic mice and as target cells. The SV40TF were grown in monolayer cultures in RPMI 1640 medium with 15 percent fetal bovine serum [FBS].

10^6 SV40TF were injected into the footpads of the isogeneic Balb/c mice. 10 days later the animals were bled; afterwards the animals were killed and the lymphnodes and spleens removed. Xenogeneic antiserum was produced by immunization of rabbits to SV40TF; the antiserum was absorbed with mouse red blood cells. The cytotoxic titer of the mouse serum determined in a dye exclusion test was less than 1 : 32, the rabbit antiserum had a cytotoxic titer of 1 : 250. The DNA-synthesis inhibition test

was performed according to a modification of the test described
by WARNATZ et al. [1]. 10^5 SV40 TF were cultivated in tube
cultures in 3 ml RPMI 1640 medium with 15 percent FBS 24 hours
prior to incubation with lymphocytes or antiserum. 10^6 or 10^7
lymphocytes or antiserum. 10^6 or 10^7 lymphocytes preincubated
with mitomycin C were added to the SV40TF-cultures. To one
part of the cultures antiserum [3 or 30 μl] was added. After 24
hours the cultures were incubated with 5 μCi ^{3}H-thymidine for
10 hours. The cultures were washed in cold RPMI-1640 medium
afterwards and the ^{3}H-thymidine incorporated into the nuclear
DNA of the SV40TF was measured in a liquid scintillation counter.
The inhibition index was calculated as

$$II = \frac{cpm_{TC + LC + antiserum}}{cpm_{TC}}$$

The microcytotoxicity test was performed according to the instructions of TAKASUGI and KLEIN [2], modified by HELL-
STRÖM et al. [3]. As target cells SV40TF were used. 200 cells
suspended in 100 μl medium were plated in each well of the microtest plates. The cells were incubated for 6^h in a gassed incubator
in order to let the target cells adhere to the bottom of the wells.
200, 2000 or 20.000 lymphocytes suspended in 200 μl of culture
medium and in controls 200 μl culture medium were added to the
wells of each row. The cytotoxicity of lymphocytes was tested in
the presence of normal mouse serum and of mouse or rabbit
antiserum to SV40TF in concentrations of 1 - 10 μl per well. The
plates were incubated in the incubator for 48^h. After that time
the test was terminated by washing the plates twice with cold
medium to remove free target cells and lymphocytes. The plates
were stained with 0.1 percent crystall violet and intact cells were
counted under an inverted microscope. The percent target cells

counted in the wells were calculated according to the formula

$$\text{percent target cells} = \frac{\text{no. of cells in test}}{\text{no. of cells in control}} \text{ x } 100$$

The results obtained with the two methods are indicated in Fig.1 and 2. In the DNA-synthesis inhibition test [Fig.1] lymphocytes from immunized mice reduce the growth rate of SV40TF. The ^{3}H-thymidine incorporation is significantly below that of SV40TF cultured without addition of immunized lymphocytes. The reduction is dependent on the amount of added lymphocytes. Mouse antiserum does not inhibit the growth of SV40TF, but it impairs the inhibiting function of lymphocytes. Xenogeneic antiserum, however, is cytotoxic for the target cells; it inhibits the DNA-synthesis of target cells and enhances the effect of lymphocytes.

The results of the microcytotoxicity test are similar. Lymphocytes of immunized mice are cytotoxic for SV40TF target cells [Fig.2]. The effect is dependent on the ratio of lymphocytes to target cells. Isogeneic mouse serum interferes with the lymphocytotoxicity; the reduction of target cells in the presence of antiserum is lower than that in the absence of antiserum. On the contrary, xenogeneic antiserum increases the cytotoxic effect of lymphocytes.

The data indicate that the microcytotoxicity test and the DNA-synthesis inhibition test are qualified for the demonstration of cellular and humoral immune reactions to tumor target cells. The result of both methods are basically in agreement. The DNA-synthesis inhibition test measures growth characteristics of the tumor cells and is dependent on a rapidly growing tumor cell system with high rates of ^{3}H-thymidine incorporation into the nuclear DNA. The microcytotoxicity test can be only applied in tumor cell systems growing in monolayer cultures; it measures

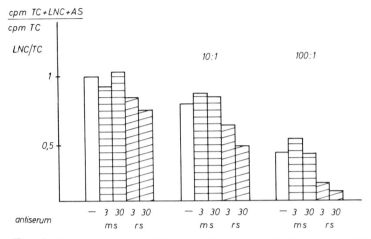

Fig. 1. Results of the DNA-synthesis inhibition test. The inhibition index for cultures of SV40TF tumor cells [TC] in the presence or absence of lymphnode cells [LNC] or antiserum is given. Mouse antiserum [ms] or rabbit antiserum [rs] to SV40TF are added in doses of 3 or 30 µl. The SV40TF are incubated without LNC, with the 10 fold or the 100 fold amount of LNC.

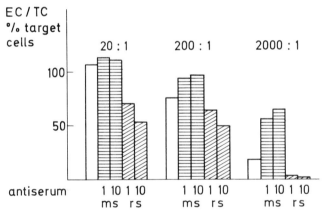

Fig. 2. Results of the microcytotoxicity test are given as % target cells counted in the test cultures in comparison to the controls without LNC or antiserum. The effector cell: target cell ratio [EC/TC] was 20:1, 200:1 or 2000:1. Mouse antiserum [ms] or rabbit antiserum [rs] were added in doses of 1 or 10 µl.

        cultures with LNC added

        cultures with LNC, mouse serum added

        cultures with LNC, rabbit serum added.

cytotoxicity, growth inhibition of the tumor cells and detachment of the tumor cells from the culture vessel. The fact that both methods determine the same reactions with different test systems explains the good correlation between their results.

References

1. WARNATZ, H., SCHEIFFARTH, F. & RÜTERS, J. [1973], Z. Krebsforsch. 79, 176

2. TAKASUGI, M. & KLEIN, E. [1970], Transplantation 9, 219

3. HELLSTRÖM, I., HELLSTRÖM, K. E., SJOGREEN, H. O. & WARNER, G. A. [1971], Int. J. Cancer 7, 1

1.7 The Leukocyte Adherence Inhibition Test for Detection of Tumor-Specific Sensitized Lymphocytes and Serum Blocking Factors

F. Lampert and E. Dietmair

I would like to present a new, simple and sensitive method to detect cell-mediated immunity of delayed [tuberculin] type. Tumor-specific immunity and its blocking by serum factors can be demonstrated by this technique in patients with malignant tumors. It is called Leucocyte Adherence Inhibition [LAI]-Test and is based upon different adherence to glass of sensitized leucocytes following antigen contact.

LAI-Test: Isolated lymphocytes and monocytes of sensitized patients are incubated with specific antigen [tuberculin or tumor extract] for 30 min. Lymphocytes are isolated from 10 ml heparinized blood by density centrifugation over a radiopaque solution [Uromiro] with specific gravity of 1076. One can harvest then - free of erythrocytes - about 1×10^6 leucocytes per ml original blood, of which 95 % are lymphocytes, 5% monocytes. To increase the percentage of monocytes or large lymphocytes to 20 - 30 %, the isolated cells are incubated in EAGLE's basal medium for 2-3 days. Those monocytes [or macrophages] are very important, as these are the cells which are altered in their glass adherence by sensitized lymphocytes after antigen contact. Drops of the cell-antigen mixture then are either given into a NEUBAUER-hemocytometer - this was the original method described by HALLIDAY and MILLER [1] for mice peritoneal cells - and following a 1 hr incubation one counts the cells in the same squares before and after immersion of the haemocytometer into HANKS' solution to obtain the percentage of adherent cells;

or - and this is our modification of the LAI-test [2] - 0,02 ml
of the cell-antigen mixture are given into prepared Coulter
counting tubes. Each of these plastic tubes contains 10 ml of
"Isoton" solution and 30 unpolished, thoroughly cleansed glass
beads, each 5 mm in diameter. The number of cells in each tube
is immediately determined with the Coulter Counter. Then the
cells in each tube are counted again after standing at room temperature for 2 hours and after one careful inversion of each tube
just before recounting [the glass beads should roll once to the
other end of the tube and then return to the old position]. Now the
percentages of adherent cells are determined for each Coulter
tube and the mean of about 10 tubes for each cell-antigen mixture
calculated. Statistical significance of the difference of the means
is examined by the **STUDENT**'s t-test.

LAI-Test and tuberculin sensitivity: Reliability of the LAI-test
was examined by the classical model of tuberculin sensitivity
[Table 1]. In tuberculin positive individuals glass adherence of
their leucocytes is significantly [from 42 to 22%, from 59 to 34%,
from 34 to 5%, from 23 to 12 %, and so on] inhibited by the in
vitro addition of tuberculin even at weak concentrations. No
significant drop of leucocyte adherence [46 to 44 %], however,
has been observed in a tuberculin negative control person. Compared with the original haemocytometer method , there is a much
lower standard deviation in our Coulter method, thus not only
saving time but also statistically being more reliable. The percentage of adherent cells is different from person to person, but
increases after cell culture for several days.

Table 1: Leucocyte adherence inhibition by tuberculin

Donor's skin test	Leuko-cyte culture [hours]	Tuber-kulin conc. [units]	Adherent cells [% of total] [Mean ± SD]	
		Haemocytometer-method		
Positive	24	-	42 ± 22	
		100	22 ± 15	$p < 0.0002$
Positive	48	-	59 ± 24	
		10	34 ± 28	$p < 0.001$
Positive	72	-	34 ± 24	
		1000	5 ± 7	$p < 0.0002$
		Coulter-method		
Negative	72	-	46 ± 6	
		10	44 ± 4	$p > 0.4$
		100	44 ± 2	$p > 0.3$
		1000	42 ± 5	$p > 0.15$
Positive	0	-	23 ± 4	
		1000	12 ± 5	$p < 0.005$
Positive	48	-	49 ± 4	
		1000	28 ± 6	$p < 0.0002$
Positive	72	-	47 ± 5	
		10	33 ± 9	$p < 0.02$
		1000	18 ± 6	$p < 0.001$
Positive	72	-	36 ± 5	
		100	22 ± 9	$p < 0.005$
		1000	22 ± 5	$p < 0.0005$

Preparation of soluble tumor extract: About 1 cm^3 of tumor is homogenized in HANKS' solution [1 part tumor to 4 parts solution] by hand with a glass homogenizer. Cell debris is separated by centrifugation for 30 min. at 1000 x g. The supernatant then is further purified by centrifugation at 100000 x g for 30 min. The clear supernatant fluid having a protein content of 1-4 mg/ml will be used as tumor antigen.

LAI-Test and tumor antigen experiments: In children with different malignant tumors leucocyte adherence inhibition was tested first by their autologous tumor extracts [Table 2]. Extracts of histologically different tumors served as controls as well as leucocytes of a healthy individual. In each case the isolated lymphocytes of the patients reacted specifically with the extracts of their own tumor by a significant LAI [28 to 18%, 37 to 33%,

24 to 17 %, 30 to 31 %]; they did not, however, react with extracts of different tumors.

Table 2:   Tumor-specific inhibition of leucocyte adherence by autologous tumor extracts

Patient [Leuco-cytes]	Tumor	Antigen extract [Tumor]	% adherent cells [Average $\pm$ SD]	
DL	Healthy	-	38 ± 2	$p > 0,25$
		LD[Neuroblastoma]	39 ± 4	
LD	Neuroblastoma	-	28 ± 2	$p < 0,0005$
		LD	18 ± 4	
		GW[Hepatocarcinoma]	27 ± 5	
HR	Nephroblastoma	-	37 ± 3	$p < 0,05$
		HR	33 ± 4	
		FXL[Neuroblastoma]	39 ± 4	
GW	Hepatocarcinoma	-	24 ± 7	$p < 0,01$
		GW	17 ± 3	
		LD[Neuroblastoma]	23 ± 2	
MP	Reticulosarcoma	-	39 ± 5	$p < 0,01$
		MP	31 ± 5	
		HS[Lymphosarcoma]	38 ± 3	

In children with neuro- and nephroblastoma it could be demonstrated that their lymphocytes reacted similarly to extracts of homologous, histologically similar tumors [Table 3]. Leucocyte adherence of patients with neuroblastoma not only is inhibited by its autologous tumor extract but also of extracts of neuroblastomas of different patients: e.g. neuroblastoma antigen FXL of a strong hormone producing tumor of a 10 year old boy caused the strongest inhibition [37 to 14%] with the lymphocytes of a 10 year old girl [SB] also having a neuroblastoma.

Table 3:   Tumor-specific inhibition of leucocyte adherence by homologous tumor extracts

Patient [Leucocytes]	Tumor	Antigen extract [Tumor]	% adherent cells Average $\pm$ SD	
RR	Neuroblastoma	-	$39 + 3$	$p<0.0005$
		LD[Neuroblastoma]	$21 + 4$	
LD	Neuroblastoma	-	$28 + 2$	$p<0.0005$
		FXL[Neuroblastoma]	$13 + 4$	
		GW[Hepatocarcinoma]	$27 + 5$	
SB	Neuroblastoma	-	$37 + 3$	$p<0.0005$
		LD[Neuroblastoma]	$22 + 5$	
		FXL[Neuroblastoma]	$14 + 4$	
LS	Neuroblastoma	-	$37 + 1$	
		LD[Neuroblastoma]	$19 + 2$	$p<0.0005$
		HR[Nephroblastoma]	$38 + 2$	
RT	Nephroblastoma	-	$53 + 4$	$p<0.0005$
		HR[Nephroblastoma]	$40 + 3$	
SW	Nephroblastoma	-	$43 + 5$	$p<0.005$
		HR[Nephroblastoma]	$32 + 7$	
		FXL[Neuroblastoma]	$41 + 3$	
GJ	Nephroblastoma	-	$39 + 2$	
		HR[Nephroblastoma]	$35 + 2$	$p<0.025$
		FXL[Neuroblastoma]	$39 + 3$	

In children with WILMS' tumor [nephroblastoma] a significant LAI could be produced with a WILMS-tumor extract which was made from a lung metastasis of a 2 year old boy; not, however, by extracts from various neuroblastomas. Neuro- and nephroblastoma seem to retain their specific antigens even in different hosts.

Table 4: Blocking of tumor-specific leucocyte adherence inhibition by serum of patients with growing tumor

Patient [Leucocytes]	Tumor	Antigen extract [Tumor]	Serum	% adherent cells [Average $\pm$ SD]	
SB	Neuroblastoma metastasizing	-	-	37 ± 3	
		-	SB	37 ± 5	
		FXL[Neuroblastoma]-		14 ± 4	
		FXL	SB	42 ± 4	$p<0.0005$
LD	Neuroblastoma no tumor	-	-	45 ± 10	
		-	LD	46 ± 5	
		LD	-	9 ± 5	
		LD	LD	14 ± 3	
		LD	RR^{+}]	39 ± 4	$p<0.0005$
SW	Nephroblastoma metastasizing	-	-	43 ± 5	
		-	SW	44 ± 4	
		HR[Nephroblastoma] -		32 ± 7	
		HR	SW	44 ± 3	$p<0.0025$
ES	Lymphosarcoma leukemic	-	-	45 ± 5	
		-	ES	42 ± 5	
		ES	-	12 ± 6	
		ES	LD	18 ± 7	$p>0.05$
		ES	ES	40 ± 5	$p<0.0005$

+] [Metast. neuroblastoma]

Table 4 exhibits an important phenomenon, i.e. the blocking effect of serum from tumor patients. Tumor specific leucocyte adherence inhibition e.g. from 37 to 14% is completely blocked [rise again to 42%] by in vitro addition of patient's serum. This reaction also seems to be very specific as serum of a patient with a different tumor [LD = neuroblastoma] cannot block the LAI [45 to 14%] in a patient with leukemic lymphosarcoma [rise only to 18% vs. 40% caused by addition of patient's own serum]. Some weeks after tumor removal in a completely tumor free state the LAI [45 to 9%] of the patient LD with neuroblastoma can only mildly be blocked by the patient's serum [rise to only 14%] as compared to the addition of serum derived from a kachectic 4 year old boy with disseminated neuroblastoma [rise to 39%].

In summary: The leucocyte adherence inhibition [LAI]-test is a simple and sensitive method which can easily be applied in clinical work. By the LAI-test one can detect not only tumor specific or antigen sensitized lymphocytes but also the blocking action of serum of the tumor patients.

References

1. HALLIDAY, W.J. & MILLER, S. [1972], Int.J.Cancer 9, 477
2. LAMPERT, F. & DIETMAIR, E., A leucocyte adherence inhibition test for cell-mediated immunity, Klin.Wochenschr. [in press]

2 Methods for Detection of Molecular Antibodies against Tumor Proteins

2.1 A Special Aspect of the Complement Fixation Test Applied to the Study of Tumors

P. Lovisetto, G. Guarini, G. Molfese and V. Biarese

In 1958, SERRA et al. [1], presented a special reaction applied to the study of tumors. Its technical modalities were similar to those of the complement fixation reactions.

Human serum was brought into contact with type 0, variety 2, whole foot-and-mouth virus in the form of a homogenated extract from artificially infected bovine tongue or guinea-pig plantar epithelium, or from a virus culture on a monostrate of bovine renal cells.

The reaction was positive [absence of haemolysis] in a large number of healthy subjects or patients with non-tumoral disease, and negative [haemolysis] in a significant percentage of patients with malignant neoplasia or haemolymphoblastosis.

Similar results were observed in the experimental animal.

Bovine tongue epithelial extracts infected with A and C foot-and-mouth virus, and their varieties, did not show the same pattern with respect to the reaction. The use of healthy bovine tongue homogenate and such viruses as those of fowl pox, Newcastle disease, swine fever, herpes simplex, parotitis, yellow fever and A, B and C type influenza was without result.

Subsequent experiments led to the employment of foot-and-mouth virus RNA instead of the whole virus. This was obtained by means of GIERER and SCHRAMM'S phenol method and presented the following chemical and physical characteristics: U.V. absorption, 240-260 nm ; biuret and diphenylamine, negative; electrophoretic mobility towards the anode, sensitivity to pyronin, negative PAS on agar, positive reaction to orcinol for values over 40 μg/ml.

Results obtained with the modified method are in line with those originally observed [2 - 8].

RNA extracted by means of the same method from healthy bovine tongue epithelium and from normal and neoplastic human and animal tissues [brain, stomach, intestine, breast, rat ascites tumor, mouse 180 sarcoma] proved inactive, as did the RNA's of Newcastle disease [obtained from virus cultures], tobacco mosaic virus [homogenates of artificially infected leaves], and commercial yeast.

The RNA of a Saccharomyces cerevisiae mutant obtained by irradiation at the University of Louvain's Cancer Institute [MAISIN and DECKERS], on the other hand, displayed a reaction activity on all fours with that of foot-and-mouth virus RNA. The physical and chemical characteristics of these two RNA's are the same, except that values in the orcinol test are as high as 150-170 μg/m for the mutant.

Method

a] Materials:

1] Fresh human serum, not heat-inactivated: this also acts as the complement.

2] Type 0, variety 2 foot-and-mouth or Saccharomyces cerevisiae virus RNA [method of GIERER and SCHRAMM].

3] Haemolytic mixture [ram red cells].

b] Reaction procedure:

Serum diluted 1:10 in 0.5 ml sodium veronal buffer [pH 7.2] + 40 μg/ml RNA in 0.3 ml of the same buffer are kept at 37°C for 30 min. 0.5 ml haemolytic mixture is added and positive and negative reactions [i.e. absence or presence of haemolysis respectively] are observed after a further 30 min. at 37°C.

Fig.1.

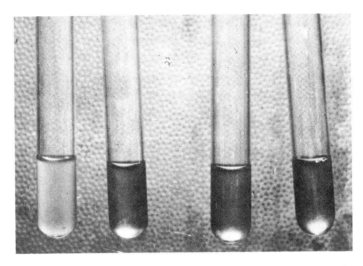

Positive reaction   Control   Negative reaction   Control
[no haemolysis]   [haemolysis]

Table 1:

	Total	Positive reaction	Negative reaction
Healthy subjects	586	83.0%[486]	17, 0%[100]
Tumor patients	904	32.3%[292]	67.7%[612]
Patients with non-tumoral diseases	1008	65.3%[659]	34.7%[349]
	2498		

Further study in the neonate and young child showed that cord blood gave a very large percent of negative reactions. This was in marked contrast to the positive reaction obtained with maternal blood withdrawn during labour.

Table 2:

	Total	Positive reaction	Negative reaction
Neonates [at term]	100	11	89
Mothers	100	89	11

As can be seen in Table 3, the reaction becomes more frequently positive with age from 6 months. After 2 yr, values are similar to those observed in the healthy adult.

Table 3:

Age	Total	Positive reaction	Negative reaction
1-6 months	40	0 % [0]	100 % [40]
6-12 months	32	43.7% [14]	56.3% [18]
1-2 years	25	56.0% [14]	44.0% [11]
2-12 years	146	82.9% [121]	17.1% [25]
	243		

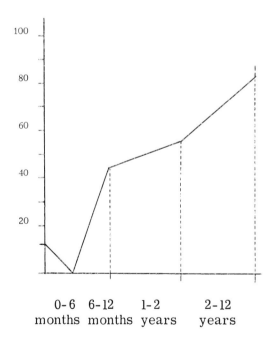

Fig. 2.
Graph showing percents of normal reactions in function of age

Electrophoresis was also done using 1% purified Difco agar in a
pH 8.4 sodium veronal buffer. Two slits were made on each slide
with Whatman 1 filter paper. Fresh, undiluted serum was brought
into contact with the pH 7.2 sodium veronal buffer for 30 min. at
37°C and placed in the top slit. A similar quantity of serum was
also brought into contact with yeast RNA in a water-bath for
30 min. at 37°C and placed in the bottom slit. The slides were
then examined electrophoretically [7-8 mA per slide; exit
voltage 130-150 volts; migration time, 75-100 min.]. Five distinct and well separated bands extending from the albumins to
the globulins were observed.

In healthy subjects, the addition of RNA resulted in the modification of a beta globulin band, whereas no changes of any kind were
observed in cancer-bearing patients.

Fig. 3.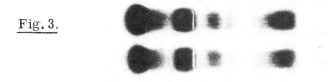

Electrophoresis of serologically positive serum from a healthy
subject. Top: serum + buffer. Bottom: serum + RNA

Fig. 4.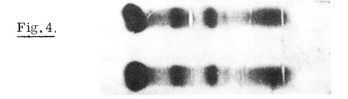

Electrophoresis of serologically negative serum from a cancer-
bearing patient. Top: serum + buffer. Bottom: serum + RNA

Results obtained in a smaller series are shown in Table 4.

Table 4:

	Total	Modification of beta globulin band	No modification
Healthy subjects	81	85.2 % [69]	14.8% [12]
Tumor patients	175	34.3 %[60]	65.7% [115]
Patients with non-tumoral diseases	187	69.0 % [129]	31.0% [58]
	443		

PEARSON's chi square test showed the non-casual nature of both
the serological and the electrophoretic data.

Two explanations may be suggested for the mechanism underlying
the serological and electrophoretic findings. In the first place,
both may be attributed to immunological interaction between a
possible serum reagent factor [factor X] and certain antigen
structures. Such a factor would thus be assumed to be present
in most healthy subjects and lacking in most cancer-bearing
patients. The pattern observed in the neonate and in very early
life lends support to this view.

Alternatively, reference may be made to findings of DECKERS
and GUARINI [9]. Using acrylamide gel electrophoresis and
immuno-electrophoresis [SCHEIDEGGER's micromethod with
$ß_1C$ /$ß_1A$ specific immunosera], these workers observed a
$ß_1C$ to $ß_1A$ transformation of the C3 complement fraction in
healthy subjects after contact with yeast RNA. This change was
absent in most patients with malignant neoplasia or haemolymphoblastosis.

References

1. SERRA,A.,GUARINI,G.,LOVISETTO,P.,CASTELLI,D. & BALZOLA,F. [1958], Nature [London] 181,622

2. SERRA,A., GUARINI,G.,GUIDETTI,E.,MAISIN,J. & DECKERS,Ch. [1965],Nature [London] 206,1264

3. MAISIN,J.,GUARINI,G.,LOVISETTO,P.,SERRA,A. & GUIDETTI,E. [1967], Bull.Acad.Roy.Med. Belgique 7,289

4. LOMBARD,A.,GUARINI,G. & DECKERS,Ch. [1967],Ann. Inst. Pasteur 137,112

5. LOVISETTO,P., MOLFESE,G.,BOGGIATTO,A.,BIARESE, V. & GUARINI,G. [1968], La Presse Méd. 76, 1327

6. GUARINI,G.,LOVISETTO,P., MOLFESE,G.,BOGGIATTO, A., BIARESE,V., MOIRAGHI RUGGENINI,A.,ERRIGO,E., MAISIN,J.,DECKERS,Ch. & VAN DUYSE,E. [1969], La Presse Méd. 77,53

7. LOVISETTO,P., MOLFESE,G., BOGGIATTO,A.,BIARESE, V.,GUARINI,G. & VISCONTI,A. [1969], La Presse Méd. 77,1383

8. NIGRO,N.,GUARINI,G.,BENSO,L.,MADON,E.,IUDICELLO, P. & JACOB,R.M. [1971], La Presse Méd. 79,227

9. DECKERS,Ch. & GUARINI,G.[1971],The third fraction of complement in healthy and cancer bearing humans,Protides Biol. Fluids, Proc. of the 18th Colloq.,Pergamon Press, Oxford - New York.

2.2 Principle and Technique of the „Lewis-3 D Test" for the Serological Diagnosis of Malignancy – A Critical Evaluation of the Results

C. C. Schneider and H. Uebel

The search for a technically simple and practicable test for cancer specific antigens in serum from patients with cancer led to the development of the so-called "Lewis-3 D test". Although it has been the subject of several reports [1, 2, 3] the test has not been widely adopted.

The present study deals first of all with the performance of the test and the preparation of reagents. The results of personal experience with the test are then summarized. From these it will be apparent why the procedure has not been accepted as a specific serological test for cancer diagnosis.

Materials and Method

In the late fifties DE CARVALHO, using halogenated hydrocarbons [fluorocarbons] as solvents, began to extract specific lipophilic constituents from tumors. These substances, which cannot be isolated by extraction with aqueous solvents, are claimed to be potential tumor antigens which can be used for the production of antibodies by immunizing horses [4, 5]. The process of fluorocarbon extraction was originally published by GESSLER in 1956 for the isolation of virus-specific nucleoproteins [6].

Figure 1 shows how so-called "antinormal sera" and "antitumor sera" were produced, first by DE CARVALHO and then by A. LEWIS [7], and how the necessary antigens were prepared. One of the materials processed by the fluorocarbon extraction method was nonmalignant human tissue, obtained from operation and amputation specimens. This "normal antigen" was injected into horses so as to produce "antinormal antibody".

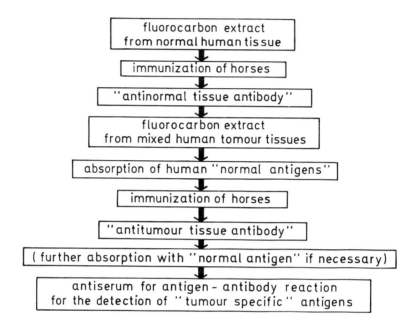

Fig. 1. Stages in the production of antisera.

These "antinormal sera" produced in horses contained antibodies against normal human proteins and were used for the absorption of normal non-tumor-specific human antigens from tumor extracts; they were also employed as one of the necessary test reagents [Reagent A] in the 3-D test [1, 2, 3].

The actual tumor antigen, also used for immunizing horses, was produced as follows. Tissue from various kinds of tumors, obtained at operations and biopsies, was homogenized and extracted in the cold with Frigen 113 and glycine buffer [pH 10.4]. This resulted in a gel-like material which was suspended in glycine buffer and mixed with the "antinormal serum" described above, so as to absorb any normal antigens still present. It was then given in a course of injections to horses in order to produce "antitumor antisera".

The "antitumor antisera" were collected by bleeding the horses at intervals and subsequently used as Reagent B for the 3-D test.

In the procedure known as the 3-D test patients'sera were used as antigen reagents and the horse sera described above as anti body reagents. Serum from horses which has been immunized with fluorocarbon extracts of non-neoplastic human tissue, either necrotic or healthy, was designated as Reagent A. It was placed in wells in an agar plate, punched out in a ring round a central well, and left for 24 hours to diffuse into the surrounding agar, in the hope that "normal antigens" in the patients'sera could thus be absorbed before it was allowed to react with the "antitumor serum". The peripheral wells were then refilled with sera from the patients under examination. These sera under test, as also control sera run at the same time, were likewise allowed to diffuse for 24 hours before the actual "antitumor serum" - termed Reagent B - was placed in the central well. [reagent B was serum from the horses which had been immunized with purified fluorocarbon extracts of human tumor tissue.] The antiserum was given a further 24 or 48 hours to diffuse from the central well and the agar plate was then scrutinized for precipitation lines.

Results

Figure 2 shows how the plates looked when tumor-positive reaction lines - as described by LEWIS - had appeared. It is a diagram of the possible precipitation lines. The individual lines are identified by letters [1].

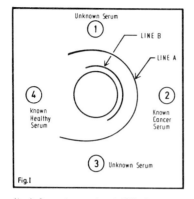
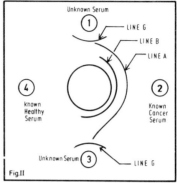

Line A – Cancer. In approximately 95 % of the cancer sera tested, one sees lines as in Figure I The nature of Line B is not understood at the present time.

Line G – Cancer. In about 5 % of known cancer sera one sees a pattern such as that in Figure II For purposes of categorization this line has been called Line G but is nevertheless interpreted as positive for cancer.

(LEWIS, A.J. a.o., Cancer Cytology Journal 1966)

Fig. 2. Diagram of the precipitation lines which may appear in the 3-D test [from LEWIS et al.].

The most conspicuous feature of Figure 2 is the very strong line A, which was noted in 95 % of sera from cancer cases. Inside this there is line B, which LEWIS was unable to identify and which is thought not to be cancer-specific. Besides line A and line B there is a line identified by the letter G. Line G is said to be found in 5 % of cancer sera.

These claims may be summarized by saying that when the test is carried out as described above there are two different precipitation lines which can be regarded as cancer-specific.

Attempts have been made to use the test to follow the kinetics of "tumor antigens" in patients' blood. This has been done by semi-quantitative assessment of the results [expressed in terms of reaction strength] obtained at intervals from cancer patients under treatment with cytostatic agents, radiotherapy or surgery. Large numbers of human sera have been screened for so-called cancer antigens; the results are summarized in Table 1 [7].

Table 1: Summary of 3-D test findings reported by LEWIS divided into correct and incorrect results.

Table 1 — Summary of Double Blind Studies
Lewis Test Correlation with Histopathology and Clinical Diagnosis

STUDY NUMBER	STUDY SOURCE	NUMBER OF PATIENTS	CANCER PATIENTS		SICK NON-CANCER OR PRESUMED CURED			HEALTHY BY PHYSICAL EXAM			TOTAL NUMBER OF SPECIMENS TESTED INCLUDING REPEATS
			T+	F—	T—	F+	F+*	T—	F+	F+*	
1	F.O.R.	153	66	8	40	1	7	31			1,143
2	M.H.	88	70	8	3	2	4	1			100
3	D.M.C.	1,736	73	16	50	7		1,589	1		1,736
4	P.D.C.	86	43	2	29	5	7				86
5	N.C.C.	188	168	20							188
6	C.R.	900	2					892	5	1	900
7	Misc. Hospitals	584	229	10	156	10	19	160			584**
8	Misc. Physicians	246	228	18							3,702
GRAND TOTALS		3.981	879	82	278	25	37	2 673	6	1	8,439
ACCURACY			$\frac{T+}{T+(+)F-}$ 91.46%		$\frac{T-}{T-(+)F+(+)F+*}=81.11\%$ $\frac{T-}{T-(+)F+}$ 91.74%			$\frac{T-}{T-(+)F+(+)F+*}=99.70\%$			

From the data in the table it will be seen that the results from sera from cancer patients were divided into true positives and false negatives, while those from non-cancer patients and healthy people were divided into false positives and true negatives. The total of 3,981 subjects was classified into cancer patients, patients with diseases other than cancer, and healthy people. Looking at the test results on sera from healthy people, we see that they were nearly all negative. In other words, in healthy people the 3-D test gave "correct negative" results in 99 %. Sera from patients with conditions other than cancer gave negative results in 81 % of cases and "false positive" results in less than 20 %. The likelihood of such false positive results is the reason why the 3-D test should not be carried out on patients with injuries, necrotic tissue lesions, fractures, gastric ulcers or recent surgical operations. The same restriction applies to patients with acute or chronic inflammatory conditions such as rheumatic fever or pneumonia.

When we look at the results derived from cancer patients it is apparent that the vast majority of them gave a "correct positive" result; calculated in comparison with the "false negatives" the figure for "correct positives" was 91 %.

Original investigations [+]

In view of the figures cited above - 91 % correct positives in sera from cancer patients, 99 % correct negatives in sera from healthy people and at least 80 % correct negatives in sera from non-cancer patients - it seemed reasonable to investigate the potentialities of the 3-D test as a method of detecting cancer-specific antigens in serum from cancer patients.

The first step was to analyze whether the two allegedly tumor-specific precipitation lines were really attributable to two tumor antigens. It soon became apparent that the precipitation band which LEWIS called Tumor Line A was due to the presence of C-reactive protein [CRP] in the patient's serum. LEWIS's other band - Tumor Line G - was due to a serum protein which was antigenically identical with fibrin or fibrinogen and therefore not cancer-specific.

It was therefore not possible to demonstrate cancer-specific antigens in serum from cancer patients by immunizing horses with fluorocarbon extracts from human cancer tissue and employing

[+]   We wish to thank Dr.med.HOYNG,Cologne, for the control serum samples, Dozent Dr. KARRER,Vienna, for numerous cancer sera and M.KASCHEL, U.HIMMEL and C.SCHUMACHER for their unfailingly reliable technical assistance. Special information and sufficient amounts of test reagents were given to us by Rand Development Corp.,Cleveland/ Ohio which were appreciated very much.

the resulting antisera in the LEWIS 3-D procedure. These findings also explain why the LEWIS 3-D test for tumor diagnosis is contraindicated in cases of hepatic cirrhosis, myocardial infarction, appendicitis, pneumonia, fractures and major injuries; it is just such patients who have raised CRP levels. Furthermore, now that the antigenic nature of the serum protein responsible for the supposed tumor line G has been identified, it is apparent why plasma gives false positive results when used instead of serum. These findings also explain why the Lewis test is today regarded as an alternative technique for the detection of CRP.

In view of the results obtained by antigenic analysis of the 3-D test, it was thought desirable to set up comparative tests with anti-CRP and antifibrinogen antisera [Behringswerke AG, Marburg/Lahn]. Table 2 summarizes the results obtained in tests carried out on nearly 2300 sera. None of the 3-D test results are included in the table, but only the positive or negative reactions with anti-CRP and anti-fibrinogen antibodies.

Table 2: Positive or negative reactions with patients' and control sera tested with precipitating anti CRP and anti-fibrinogen antibodies.

	Serum proteins detected by:				number of sera
	Anti-CRP antibody		Antifibrinogen antibody		
	+	−	+	−	
Clinically confirmed cancer cases	159 80%	40 20%	104 52%	95 48%	199
Inoperable cancer cases	15 94%	1 6%	11 69%	5 31%	16
Cancer cases after operation or radio-therapy	35 58%	25 42%	5 8%	55 92%	60
Inflammatory and necrotic conditions	66 79%	18 21%	21 25%	63 75%	84
Pregnancy and puerperium	20 80%	5 20%	4 16%	21 84%	25
Clinically healthy people	209 12%	1697 88%	6 0.3%	1900 99.7%	1906

The results summarized above show that the incidence of positive reactions with both antibodies was far higher in sera from cancer patients than in sera from patients who were free from cancer.

Discussion

Although there are still no tests for genuinely tumor-specific antigens, it seems worthwhile to report the results obtained in this study. The CRP values in cancer patients and the "fibrinogen values" in both cancer and non-cancer patients deserve special attention. It can perhaps be concluded from these findings that the demonstration - technically not a matter of any difficulty - of antigen-antibody reactions between the patient's serum in one well and anti-CRP or antifibrinogen antibody in other wells raises serious suspicion of cancer. Whether perhaps MANCINI radial immunodiffusion plates should be used for this purpose [Fig. 3] is open to discussion.

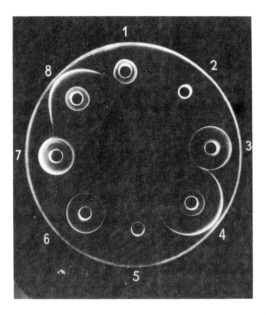

Fig. 3. Precipitation rings given by sera from cancer patients in a MANCINI plate containing anti-CRP and anti-fibrinogen antibodies.

1. Human plasma
2. Negative human control serum
3. Serum from case of carcinoma of tongue
4. Serum from case of sarcoma of nasal sinuses
5. Negative human control serum
6. CRP-positive control serum
7. Serum from a case of carcinoma of nasal sinuses
8. Serum from case of carcinoma of nasopharynx.

The simultaneous appearance of two precipitation rings is at least strongly suggestive of cancer, because these rings represent tissue breakdown within the tumor and fibrinolysis caused by it. The work revealed one interesting finding, namely that squamous carcinomas arising from mucosal surfaces [e.g. carcinoma of the tongue, pharynx, oesophagus, larynx, vagina and vulva] gave positive results in 90% of cases. This finding requires confirmation.

Summary

The method known as the Lewis test or 3-D test for demonstrating cancer-specific antigens in the serum of cancer patients was based on the use of antisera produced by immunizing horses with fluoro-carbon extracts of human tumor tissue.

It was not possible to confirm the high proportion of "correct positive" and "correct negative" results reported elsewhere. In the course of the present work it became apparent that the main precipitation line is due to C-reactive protein and for this reason the Lewis test is now regarded as a test for the latter.

However, a high proportion of sera from cancer patients reacted with both anti-CRP and antifibrinogen antibodies. The technique is simple and - although nonspecific - might be of some value for the serological detection of cancer or for follow-up.

References

1. LEWIS, A. J., RAND, H. J. & AYRE, J. E. [1966], Cancer Cytol. J. 6/2, 55

2. AYRE, J. E. et al. [1967], Cancer Cytol. J. 7, 1

3. KILLIAN, H. A., CAHILL, J. J. & FARRINGTON, D. L. et al. [1968], J. Industrial Med. & Surg. 37, 2

4. DeCARVALHO, S. [1960], J. Lab. Clin. Med. 56, 333

5. DeCARVALHO,S.[1963],Cancer Cytol.J. <u>16</u>, 306

6. GESSLER,A.E.,BENDER,C.E. & PARKINSON,M.C.[1955-1956],Trans.N.Y.Acad.Sci. <u>18</u>, 701

7. LEWIS,A.J.,"The Lewis Test" - A serologic test for cancer detection and therapeutic follow-up, in Scientific Information from Lewis[3-D]Test, Inc.Box 20187 Shaker Heights,Ohio 44120,USA·

3 Methods for Detection of Tumor Cell Surface Antigens

3.1 The Preparation and Application of Hybrid Antibody for the Detection of Tumor-Specific Cell Surface Antigens

H. Gelderblom

Conventional transmission electron microscopy [EM] is based on the different electron scattering intensities of the components in the object under investigation. The electron beam is weakened at places of high mass density, while its intensity is only slightly diminished in regions of low mass concentration. This difference gives rise to contrast, and from this phenomenon conclusions can be drawn with regard to shape and the composition of objects. In principle, conventional electron microscopy is describing only the presence and distribution of physico-chemical entities, namely the arrangement of different groups of atoms of high atomic number in the specimen.

The electron density of biological specimens consisting mainly of carbon, hydrogen, oxygen and sulfur is often so weak that it has to be increased by artificial contrasting. The chemical groups are detected and discriminated by their varying affinity to different electron dense staining agents, e.g. heavy metal atoms. Thus, dark and lucent spots are observed on the microscope screen after staining. These correspond to regions of artificial high or low mass concentration in the specimen.

Antigenic changes on the cell surface that occur in the course of malignization of a normal cell are of great theoretical and practical interest. Conventional EM alone does not allow the detection of such antigens. Corresponding antibodies are large enough to be detected by EM. However, without artificial contrasting, the antibody itself does not display sufficient electron scattering intensity to be detectable. Therefore it is necessary to label it with an electron dense marker permitting localization. By binding labeled antibody of known specificity to biological specimens, it is possible to locate the respective antigens bound in the antigen-antibody complex.

In 1954, FARRANT [1] proposed horse spleen ferritin as a suitable marker for EM and in 1959, SINGER [2] prepared covalent ferritin-antibody conjugates using bivalent diisocyanates as the coupling agents. Such conjugates were first used in 1960 by C. MORGAN and his group [3] for the detection of influenza virus structural antigens. The immunoferritin technique was later modified by using heavy atoms [Hg : PEPE [4]; U : STERNBER-GER, [5]] or enzyme-substrate complexes [AVRAMEAS [6], KURSTAK [7], STERNBERGER [8]] as marker molecules.

Unfortunately the covalent ferritin-antibody conjugates show a decreased specific activity. Since the diisocyanates react with every lysine residue they produce a certain amount of aggregation. More important, the specific binding regions of the antibody are often sterically hindered. In addition the coupling conditions destroy part of the antibody activity. Therefore at most 10 percent of the initial activity of the native antibody is available in the final conjugate.

These drawbacks led HÄMMERLING et al. in 1968 [9] to use hybrid antibody [HY-AB] for binding the electron dense marker to the antigen-antibody complex. HY-AB represent divalent IgG fragments with two binding regions of different specificity. These heterodimers bind the antigen to one recognition site and the marker to the second site.

HY-AB is prepared according to NISONOFF and RIVERS [10]. HÄMMERLING [9] and AOKI [11] were the first to use HY-AB in immune EM for the demonstration of cell surface antigens. HY-AB have several advantages, compared to the commonly used covalent conjugates, e.g. absence or at least diminished unspecific labeling and better resolution, due to the defined dimensions and the immunological binding of the reagent. These characteristics led us to use HY-AB in locating and differentiating tumor virus induced cell surface antigens in the avian RNA tumor virus [ATV] system [for review see BAUER [12]; VOGT [13]; VIGIER [14]]. In the following chapters I will describe first in detail the preparation of the immunoreagents. This will be followed by a brief outline of the principal results obtained by applying HY-AB to the search for tumor specific surface antigens.

Ferritin

This iron storage protein [Fig. 1] is found widely in vertebrates, plants and fungi and its synthesis can be induced in vitro under appropriate tissue culture conditions. The molecule has a diameter of about 100 - 120 Å and is characterized by its high iron content of about 20% [15]. Up to 4.000 iron atoms per molecule are contained in a micellar core 60 Å in diameter and result in a high electron scattering potential in spite of the relatively low atomic weight of Fe [=56] [16]. Ferritin has a molecular weight varying from 600,000 - 750,000 daltons depending on the amount of iron, while the iron-depleted protein shell, called apoferritin has a MW of 465,000 daltons [17].

Isolation and purification of ferritin:

The purification is done following the procedure of VOGT et al. [18]. Two or more fresh horse spleens [about 2 kg] are well minced and suspended in 2 volumes of cold glass-distilled water.

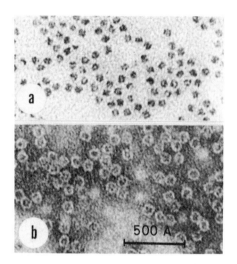

Fig. 1. Electron micrographs of horse spleen ferritin isolated as described in this chapter. Both preparations consist of pure ferritin molecules with the electron dense centers exhibiting some substructure. Without contrasting only the central iron containing core is revealed [Fig. 1a]. After negative staining with 2 percent silicotuncstic acid pH 7.0, the protein shell is also visible [Fig. 1b] Magnification : x 400,000.

After stirring vigorously for 4 hrs at $4^{\circ}C$ to lyse the cells, the suspension is centrifuged at 3.000 rpm for 20 min. The supernatant is collected and heated slowly to $80^{\circ}C$ over a period of 4 hrs under continous stirring. By this treatment most of the proteins will denature and precipitate. They are removed by low speed centrifugation, while the heat resistant supernatant is precipitated by 28 percent ammonium sulfate [w/v]. The brown precipitate contains ferritin and is contaminated with 20 - 50 percent apoferritin. It is suspended in glass-distilled water, thoroughly dialysed against distilled water for 2 days to remove free sulfate ions and then centrifuged 2 times at 3.000 rpm for 30 min to eliminate larger aggregates.

Due to the difference in molecular weight, the heavier ferritin sediments faster than apoferritin. Therefore, the low speed supernate is subjected to ultracentrifugation in a Spinco rotor 30. After 6 hrs at 30,000 rpm, the yellow-brown supernatant is decanted and the black sediment [ferritin] is resuspended in distilled water by vigorous pipetting. After 3-4 repeated centrifugations of the resuspended ferritin pellets, a relatively pure monomeric ferritin preparation [Fig. 1] is obtained that contains only traces of apoferritin. Due to the absence of the iron core, the latter is detected in the EM after negative staining by its electron transparent center. Only small amounts of ferritin aggregates are observed. The dimer, called ß-ferritin represents [19] less than 10 percent, and is present also naturally without centrifugation. Recrystallization to separate ferritin from apoferritin is not necessary since the purity of this ferritin preparation is sufficient for immune-EM. The concentration of ferritin can be determined by its absorbancy at 440 nm. 1 OD unit measured in a 1 cm cell represents a concentration of 650 μg ferritin/ml [A. VOGT, personal communication, 1970].

Ferritin stocks are stored in sealed glass ampoules after sterile filtration [Millipore, 0,45 μm] at concentrations of up to 100 mg/ml.

Hybrid Antibodies

HY-AB for immunoferritin labeling are prepared in vitro by combining IgG split products, i.e. monovalent Fab' fragments of two different specificities directed either against the ferritin marker or against the antigen to be labeled. The choice of the animal species to supply the immune sera is important, since even in the IgG class of antibody there exists a high structural diversity [N. HILSCHMANN, personal communication]. One of the most simply constructed class of IgG molecules is found in high amount in the 7 S fraction of the rabbit. The dimeric structure is held together in its two-fold symmetry plane by one single disulfide bond [20]. This bond can be effectively split by reduction and reassociated by oxidation as shown in Fig. 2. This Figure summarizes the nomenclature and some biochemical and structural properties

Rabbit JgG Antibody (7S)

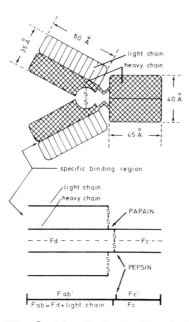

Fig. 2. Morphological and biochemical properties of rabbit IgG. The upper model adapted from the work of VALENTINE and GREEN [34] demonstrates ultrastructural properties. The scheme below gives additional details of the biochemically evaluated substructures and their nomenclature according to PUTNAM [35].

of the rabbit IgG. Guinea pig IgG, for example, is held together by 3 disulfide bonds [21], which can be split only by much higher concentrations of the disulfide reagent [22], and this may also affect other intra-chain disulfide bonds of the monomeric Fab'.

Difficulty in the preparation of HY-AB arises from the fact that even in highly immunized animals the fraction of specifically reacting antibody is rather low, in general not more than 20 percent. If one oxidizes mixtures of specific and non-specific Fab' fragments, one obtains besides other reaggregates, a high proportion of heterodimeric F $[ab']_2$, which are composed of one specific site and one nonspecific site. These dimers are able to combine only with one of the antigenic sites in which we are interested, either the marker or the antigen. For effective immune labeling, therefore, a high proportion of specifically reacting heterodimers is necessary and this is achieved only after removal or at least drastic reduction of the nonspecific antibody fractions by using immunoadsorbent techniques.

HY-AB can be applied in a direct labeling procedure as shown in Fig. 3a. However, the indirect method has several advantages, one of which is the availability of the respective sera. In the following sections a brief outline is given of the prerequisites and the techniques necessary for the preparation of a HY-AB directed against chicken IgG and ferritin, respectively. When HY-AB are applied in the indirect technique, as demonstrated schematically in Fig. 3b, the use of any chicken immune serum is suitable.

Direct (a) and indirect (b) hybrid antibody technique

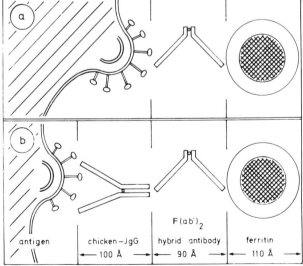

Fig. 3. Diagram of the direct [a] and the indirect [b] HY-AB technique.

Sera

Six months old rabbits are injected subcutaneously at several sites
with either 4 mg ferritin or 10 mg chicken IgG emulsified in 1 ml
of a mixture of equal parts of antigen and FREUND's incomplete
adjuvant.

I.v. booster injections of 2 mg ferritin or 4 mg chicken IgG are
given after 6 to 8 weeks on three consecutive days. In addition
4 mg chicken IgG with adjuvant is injected subcutaneously on the
first day of booster. Animals are bled on the 5th and 8th or 9th
day after the beginning of the booster and the sera are stored
frozen at -20° until further use.

Preparation of rabbit IgG

Purification of rabbit IgG is achieved in a three step method.
After removal of macromolecular proteins by precipitation during dialysis, the γ-globulins of the antisera are salt-precipitated,
followed by isolation of the IgG fractions on ion-exchange columns.

Sera of different specificity are processed separately. About 50
ml of antiserum is dialyzed for 24 hrs in the cold against several
changes of 40 volumes of 0.0025 M phosphate buffer pH 7.0. The
resulting precipitate is removed by centrifugation at 3,000 g for
10 min. For isolation of γ-globulins, two volumes of 25 percent
sodium sulfate [w/v] in phosphate buffered saline [PBS] are
added dropwise to the supernate with constant stirring at room
temperature. A white precipitate forms. Following addition of
the sodium sulfate, the solution is stirred gently for 1 hr and
then centrifuged at room temperature for 10 min at 3.000 g. The
precipitate is collected and dissolved in a volume of PBS equivalent to 1/5 of the initial serum volume. This slightly opalescent
solution contains the γ-globulins and contaminating serum pro-

teins, mainly albumin. Following dialysis at 4^oC for 24 hrs a-
gainst 4 changes of 0,015 M phosphate buffer, pH 8.0, the solution
is checked for the absence of residual sulfate ions by the addition
of 1 percent barium chloride at acid pH. The IgG fractions are
then isolated by DEAE-cellulose column chromatography. The
height of the bed volume is 5 times its diameter. The columns
are preequilibrated with at least 2 volumes of the eluting 0.015 M
phosphate buffer pH 8.0 and operated under a hydrostatic pressure of about 50 cm at room temperature. Flow rates should not
exeed 100 ml/h/cm^2. Under these conditions rabbit IgG, in contrast to all other serum constituents, will not adsorb to the DEAE
cellulose and appears in the first column volume of elution buffer.
Absorbancy at 280 nm is determined and peak fractions are
pooled. The IgG pool is checked for purity by immunodiffusion
analysis and immunoelectrophoresis. After dialysis against PBS,
IgG can be stored at -20^oC for indefinite periods of time. It
should be mentioned that this simple and rapid purification
scheme is useful for rabbit, goat and human IgG. To isolate
chicken and mouse IgG, the salt precipitation is followed by molecular sieve chromatography.

Preparation of hybrid antibodies

General outline: Rabbit IgG with specificity for ferritin or
chicken IgG is split by pepsin treatment to obtain F[ab']$_2$ fragments. The specific F[ab']$_2$ are then isolated by use of the respective immunoadsorbents. Specific F[ab']$_2$ fragments will be
bound to the immunoadsorbent and after removal of the nonspecific F[ab']$_2$ and other constituents of the pepsin digest, they
can be eluted by buffers at low pH. Equal amounts of rabbit
F[ab']$_2$ specific for chicken IgG and ferritin are mixed and split

by reduction of their inter heavy-chain disulfide bond. After removal of the reducing agent and under oxidizing conditions, the majority
of the monovalent Fab' will recombine [Fig. 4]. In this process

Preparation of Hybrid Antibody

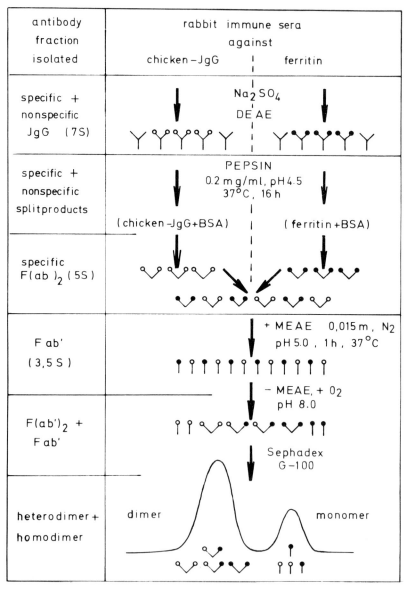

Fig. 4. Flow diagram of preparation of HY-AB.

a nearly random distribution of divalent reassociation products [9, 22] is observed, i.e. about 50 percent of the desired HY-AB, with the remaining 50 percent consisting of homodimers and a small fraction of monovalent unrecombined Fab'. The homodimer and the monovalent Fab' directed against chicken IgG will compete with the HY-AB in the labeling reaction for the chicken IgG already bound to the cell. Therefore, a further purification step is necessary. The residual monovalent Fab' is removed by molecular sieve chromatography, while the presence of the homodimers is tolerated since it does not affect the results. In principle, however, the isolation of a pure HY-AB is possible by successive treatments with chicken IgG and ferritin immunoadsorbents.

Procedure

600 mg portions of isolated IgG directed against ferritin and chicken-IgG respectively are dialyzed against 0,1 M acetate buffer, pH 4.5, for 6 hrs. The concentration of the antibody is then determined spectrophotometrically at 260 and 280 nm by the method of WARBURG and CHRISTIAN [23] and the protein concentrations are adjusted with 0.1 M acetate buffer pH 4.5 to 10 mg/ml. 6 ml of this solution is placed in an incubator at $37^\circ C$, flushed with nitrogen to replace oxygen, and 12 mg pepsin is added to a final concentration of 2 mg per 10 mg of IgG. The mixture is incubated with stirring for 16 hrs at $37^\circ C$. The reaction is stopped by adjusting the pH of the digest to about 7.0 with 1 M Na_2HPO_4 and lowering the temperature to $4^\circ C$. The

digest is then dialyzed for 3 hrs against PBS and concentrated to about 20 mg/ml by evaporation using a cold blowing fan while remaining in the dialysis tubing.

The isolation of specifically reacting $F[ab']_2$ by immunoadsorption is achieved according to the procedure of AVRAMEAS and TERNYNCK [24]. The immunoadsorbents are copolymers of chicken IgG or ferritin, glutaraldehyde-crosslinked with BSA. They are polymerized at a concentration of 50 mg protein/ml under acidic conditions as described in detail below.

1. Chicken IgG-BSA immunoadsorbent:
700 mg chicken IgG in 20 ml PBS is mixed with 300 mg crystallized BSA and stirred in an ERLENMEYER flask. The pH of the solution is adjusted to pH 5.5 - 6.0 by the addition of 1 M KH_2PO_4. 100 mg glutaraldehyde in 4 ml distilled water is then added dropwise with gentle shaking or stirring at room temperature. Thereby the mixture becomes cloudy and viscous and after 20 min without stirring it represents a slightly yellow solidified gel.

2. Ferritin-BSA immunoadsorbent:
400 mg ferritin and 1,600 mg crystallized BSA are mixed in 40 ml of 0.1 M acetate buffer pH 5.0. Then 200 mg glutaraldehyde in 8 ml distilled water is added dropwise with stirring at room temperature. Thorough gelification occours after 10 hrs at $4^\circ C$.

The antigen-BSA copolymers have to be purified before use, i. e. uncrosslinked proteins have to be removed by repeated washings at different pH conditions. This is achieved by suspending the gel in PBS and homogenizing the suspensions by a few gentle strokes in a DOUNCE homogenizer followed by repeated washings of the homogenate with PBS and centrifugation at 3,000 g for 20 min. The supernatant of each step is monitored spectrophotometrically. OD_{280} will never reach zero, because some depolymerization always takes place. When the absorbancy is below 0.05 OD_{280}, the polymer is washed several times with 0.1 M glycine buffer pH 2.4 until OD_{280} 0.005 or less is reached. After resuspending the polymer in PBS the remaining free aldehyde groups are blocked by addition of 0.1 percent hydroxy-ammonium-chloride and 1 percent normal rabbit serum for 20 min at room temperature. After three final washes with PBS and determination of the available binding capacities by reacting a sample with specific amounts of antibody, the adsorbents are ready for use. Working with slightly subequivalent concentrations of specific antibody is recommended. Between 5 and 10 percent of the crosslinked antigen in the immunoadsorbents seems to be accessible and able to bind the respective antibody.

About 10 ml of the pretested adsorbent are gently mixed with a suitable amount of neutralized pepsin-digested IgG and left for 30 min at room temperature with occasional shaking. After centrifugation at 3,000 g and 4°C for 20 min, the clear supernatant containing unbound proteins is removed and the volume, the protein content, and the residual antibody activity is determined. The adsorbent is washed 4 to 6 times with PBS with low speed centrifugation until the OD_{280} of the supernatant is less than 0.05.

Elution of specifically adsorbed F[ab']₂ from the adsorbent is achieved also in a batch procedure at 4°C. An equal volume of 0.1 M glycine buffer pH 2.4, is added to the adsorbent and the mixture is carefully adjusted to pH 2,4 with 0.1 N HCl. After centrifugation for 10 min at 3,000 g, the desorbed antibody fragments are found in the supernatant. This elution is repeated 3 to 5 times. The supernatant is rapidly neutralized by addition of

1 M Na_2HPO_4 and dialyzed for 2 hrs against PBS. Since the concentration of the eluted specific F [ab']$_2$ is in the range of only 1 - 2 mg/ml in the first eluate and considerably less in the following ones, these fractions are concentrated in dialysis bags by evaporation using a fan. This procedure is interrupted after each twofold concentration step by dialysis against PBS. By this method one achieves 6 - 8 fold concentration and 90 percent recovery of biologically active F[ab']$_2$ fragments. To concentrate volumes of 1 ml or less smaller dialysis tubing is used with Aquacide [CALBIOCHEM] for dehydration rather than a fan.

For the hybridization reaction equal amounts [at least 10 mg] of specific F[ab']$_2$ are used. In a typical experiment 40 mg each of both kinds of F[ab']$_2$ are mixed under nitrogen and adjusted to a concentration of 10 mg/ml in 8 ml of 0.1 M acetate buffer, pH 5.0. Nitrogen is used to flush the flask before 0.8 ml of the reducing agent, 2-mercaptoethylamine-HCl is added. This chemical is prepared immediatly before use under nitrogen as a 0.15 M solution in 0.1 M acetate buffer pH 5.0. The tube is sealed and incubated for 1 hr at 37°C to split the bivalent F[ab']$_2$. To remove mercapto-ethanol-amine the resulting mixture of monovalent F[ab'] fragments is passed through a column [2 x 30 cm] of AG-50 W cation exchange resin, pre-quilibrated with 0.1 M acetate buffer, pH 5. The effluent is collected monitoring A_{280}, and the pH of the fractions is raised to 8.0 by 1 M Na_2HPO_4. The mixture is stirred gently for 3 hrs in an oxygen atmosphere to allow dimerization of the monovalent Fab'. After dialysis for 1 hr against 0.05 M PBS it is concentrated 4 - 5 fold by evaporation and Aquacide dehydration. To separate the fraction of non-reassociated Fab', the mixture is applied to a Sephadex G-100 column and eluted with PBS [Fig. 5]. The dimer fraction is obtained in the first peak near to the void volume.

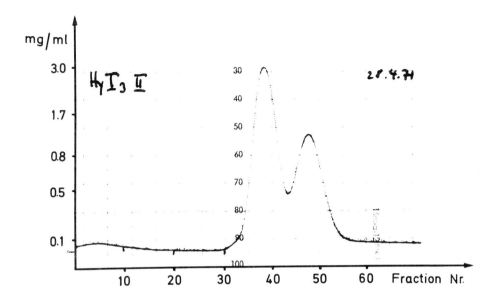

Fig. 5. Separation of reassociated dimers from the Fab′ fraction by molecular sieve chromatography on Sephadex G-100. A
Pharmacia K 15/90 column, 15 mm in diameter and 85 cm in
length, was used and 40 mg of the reoxidized mixture were
applied in a volume of 3,5 ml. Elution was with PBS under a
hydrostatic pressure of 21 cm H_2O and a flow rate of 115 ml/hr.
Transmission of the effluent is monitored at 277 μm wavelength.
Protein content of individual fractions was determed afterwards
by measuring A 260/280.

The yield is about 40 percent of the initial input of specific $F[ab′]_2$,
i.e. about 30 mg. The second peak, consisting of non-recombined
monomers, is submitted to further cation exchange chromatography after pH adjustment to 5.0, followed by reoxidation and
molecular sieve chromatography. This will yield another 5 percent reassociated $F[ab′]_2$. Protein concentration and volume of
the dimer fractions is determined and then HY-AB is stored at
-20°C without detectable loss of activity for extended periods of
time.

Application of Hybrid Antibody

HY-AB was used to investigate cells for the appearance of virus-induced cell membrane alterations. Chicken cells were preinfected with different types of avian RNA tumor viruses [ATV], namely with leukosis viruses that are able to productively infect chicken fibroblasts without concomitant transformation of the virus producing cell, and sarcoma viruses giving rise to virus production and transformation.

The immunoreagent was used in an indirect technique [Fig. 3 b]. It was hoped that immune sera from virus infected and / or tumor-bearing chickens would not only contain virus-neutralizing antibody but also antibody directed against tumor specific surface antigens if such antigens exist.

Labeling reaction

ATV infected monolayer cultures are prefixed with cold 0.5 percent glutaraldehyde in MILLONIG's buffer [25] for 5 min at $4^{\circ}C$. After 2 washes with cold PBS containing 5 percent fetal calf serum [FCS], the cells are incubated in situ with virus-neutralizing chicken sera in a 1 : 10 to 1 : 120 dilution at $25^{\circ}C$ for 20 min. This is followed by two washes with PBS-FCS before HY-AB is added that was previously diluted in the same buffer to 0.05 to 0.2 mg/ml. The cells are incubated again for 20 min at $25^{\circ}C$ and then washed two times. Ferritin is added in a concentration of 0.1 mg/ml for another 20 min incubation. Finally the cells are washed 3 times to remove unbound ferritin. They are then fixed with cold 2.5 percent glutaraldehyde in MILLONIG's buffer without sucrose for 30 min.

Electron microscopy

After postfixation with 1 percent cold osmium tetroxide in
MILLONIG's buffer the cells are dehydrated by graded ethanol
solutions, and stained with 1 percent uranyl acetate in 70 percent
ethanol for 1 hr at $20^{o}C$. The cultures are embedded in Epon 812
[26] according to published techniques [27]. Infiltration by pro-
pylene oxide is omitted because this solvent solubilizes the plastic petri dishes used for cell cultures. After polymerization for
two days at $60^{o}C$, the cells together with the Epon layer can be
easily detached from the dish if the thickness of the polymer does
not exceed 3 mm. Ultrathin sections 400-500 Å in thickness are
cut with glass knives on an Ultrotome I type ultramicrotome and
screened without additional staining in a Siemens Elmiskop I or
101 type microscope.

Characteristics of the HY-AB labeling

The immunological binding between the constituents of the reaction chain, i.e. antigen, chicken immune IgG, HY-AB, and
ferritin marker, results in defined and constant labeling dimensions. The resolution of this technique is in the range of 50 Å
and thus at least two times higher than the resolution obtained
with conventional covalent conjugates. This is demonstrated
clearly by a virus particle observed in the process of maturation
at the cell membrane [Fig. 6 a in comparison to Fig. 3]. Ferritin
is observed in different distances surrounding part of the viral
surface. The short distance found near the base of the budding
particle results from virus envelope [Ve] antigen observed just
in the moment of penetration of the viral "unit" membrane. At
the upper part of the virion the respective Ve antigenicity is
already located at the end of viral surface projections that can
directly be demonstrated by other EM techniques [28]. Mature

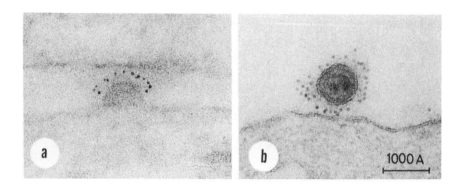

Fig. 6. Electron micrograph of immunoferritin labeled ATV.
The budding particle maturating at the cell membrane exhibits
uneven distance of the ferritin marker [a] while mature ATV
show always a complete and symmetric corona [b].
Magnification: x 150,000.

particles released from the cell display a complete ferritin corona.
This labeling is strongly virus-type-specific [29].

Labeling of the cell surface has also been observed. Utilizing
respective chicken immune sera, this cell surface reaction was
found to be due to the presence of virus envelope antigen [see
KURTH et al.; these Proceed.]. In addition, virus transformed
chicken cells display another type of antigen. It is demonstrable
only after incubation with chicken sera directed against sarcoma
viruses. This antigen is group-specific, in that all chicken sarcoma viruses induce the same kind of surface determinant independent of the envelope antigenicity of the transforming virus.
Since it is not observed on the virion itself, it is called tumor
specific cell surface antigen [TSSA] [29, 30, see also KURTH et
al. ; these Proceed.]. TSSA can also be demonstrated by several
immunological techniques on ATV transformed mammalian cells
[31, 32]. TSSA do not seem to represent one of the major virus

structural components. However, there exists some evidence
that TSSA are virus-specific in the sense that they are virus-
coded [for details, see KURTH et al.; these Proceed.].

Distribution of membrane antigens

Virus envelope antigen and TSSA were demonstrated on all parts
of the cell perimeter without a sharp delineation of labeled regions.
The distance of the ferritin from the "unit" membrane of the cell
was in the case of both antigens, 210 ± 10 Å and about 50 Å less
than the marker-membrane distance observed on the virion. This
means that the cell associated virus envelope antigen is incorporated into the cell membrane instead of residing on surface
projections. The biological implications of these antigens will be
discussed in detail by KURTH et al., these Proceedings.

Discussion of the labeling technique

The specific usefullness of the HY-AB is based on its immunological binding between antigen and marker. Therefore this method
results in well defined labeling dimensions in contrast to conventional covalent conjugates. However, since the HY-AB is a
heterodimer [with two binding regions of different specificity]
the immunological binding in certain cases may be too weak and
unreliable [22] presumably due to low avidity of the antibody
used.

On the other hand, it may well be that the monovalent binding
is reinforced in some instances in a way that two or more HY-AB
bind to one ferritin or to one antigen thus rendering the label
more stabile by crosslinking.
Because of the several-step incubation, the HY-AB labeling
technique is not well adapted for the demonstration of intracel-
lular antigens. Its domain is the search for antigenic cell surface

components. And for this purpose the indirect method demonstrated in Fig. 3 b has several advantages over the direct.

[1] A variety of antisera from one species can be used with one HY-AB [2]. The preparation of immunoadsorbents for isolation of specific antibody [fragments] is facilitated because immunoglobulins for the preparation of immunoadsorbents are by far more readily available than, for example, virus envelope antigen that would be necessary for the purification of specific chicken IgG to be used in the direct HY-AB technique [Fig. 3 a].

A brief and cautious fixation prior to labeling the cell surface is recommended for several reasons. [1] It preserves the fine structure of the cell. [2] The ferritin pattern represents the natural and actual distribution of antigen, since fixed cells are unable to react by phygocytosis, i.e. engulfment of the immuno-reagents. Furthermore, any membrane antigens that are mobile in vivo according to the fluid mosaic model proposed by SINGER [33] are immobilized on prefixed cells. Thus, no map-like distribution or aggregation of membrane antigens by the indirect labeling procedure can be observed.

The choice and the purity of the chemicals used for prefixation is critical, since notable inactivation of the antigens is commonly observed. It is necessary to screen glyoxal, glutardialdehyde and other aldehydes in different samples from different manufacturers for the best preservation of the antigen under study. Finally, the addition of 5 percent FCS or albumin to the immunoreagents and to the washing fluid results in more specific immune labeling, aids in covering unreacted aldehyde groups after prefixation, and efficiently diminishes non-specific reactions.

Summary

Immunoferritin labeling is the method of choice for the individual demonstration of antigenic molecules. The conventional ferritin technique, however, making use of chemically bound ferritin-antibody conjugates has certain limitations. The present paper deals with a more sensitive immunoferritin technique, the hybrid antibody method, which is based strictly on the specific immunological binding of the reactants, i.e. between antigen and antibody and between antibody and ferritin marker. Properties of horse spleen ferritin, antibody and hybrid antibody and detailed methods of isolation and preparation are described. Special reference is made to the application of the hybrid antibody technique in the demonstration of cell surface antigens. Finally, the advantages and limitations of the hybrid antibody technique are discussed and general recommendations are given for successful immune labeling.

Acknowledgements

The present work was performed mainly at the Max-Planck-Institut für Virusforschung in Tübingen: the author is grateful to Professor W. SCHÄFER for his steady interest and to Dr.H. FRANK for providing excellent electron microscope working conditions. I am indebted to Professor H.BAUER, Berlin, for his encouragement, support, and valuable discussions, to Dr.R. KURTH and Dr.K.F.WATSON for critically reviewing the manuscript, and to Mrs.L.KÖHLER for her competent photographic work.

References

1. FARRANT, J. F. [1954], Biochim. Biophys. Acta 13, 569

2. SINGER, S. J. [1959], Nature [London] 183, 1523

3. MORGAN, C., SHU, K. C., RIFKIND, R. A., KNOX, A. W. & ROSE, H. M. [1961], J. Exp. Med. 114, 825

4. PEPE, F. A. [1961], J. Biophys. Biochem. Cytol. 11, 515

5. STERNBERGER, L. A., DONATI, E. J. & WILSON, C. E. [1963], J. Histochem. Cytochem. 11, 48

6. AVRAMEAS, S. [1970], Int. Rev. Cytol. 27, 349

7. KURSTAK, E. [1971], in Methods in Virology V, p. 423 [eds. Maramorosch, K. and Koprowski, H.].

8. STERNBERGER, L. A. [1967], J. Histochem. Cytochem. 15, 139

9. HÄMMERLING, U., AOKI, T., DE HARVEN, E., BOYSE, E. A. & OLD, L. J. [1968], J. Exp. Med. 128, 1461

10. NISONOFF, A. & RIVERS, M. M. [1961], Arch. Biochem. Biophys. 93, 460

11. AOKI, T., BOYSE, E. A., OLD, L. J., DE HARVEN, E., HÄMMERLING, U. & WOOD, H. A. [1970], Proc. Nat. Acad. Sci. USA 65, 569

12. BAUER, H. [1970], Zbl. Vet. -Med. B 17, 582

13. VOGT, P. K. [1965], Adv. Virus Res. 11, 293

14. VIGIER, Ph. [1970], Progr. Med. Virol. 12, 240

15. LAUFBERGER, V. [1937], Bull. Soc. Chim. Biol. 19, 1575

16. FISCHBACH, F. A. & ANDEREGG, J. W. [1965], J. Molecular Biol. 14, 458

17. ROTHEN, A. [1944], J. Biol. Chem. 152, 679

18. VOGT, A., BOCKHORN, H., KOZIMA, K. & SASAKI, M. [1968], J. Exp. Med. 127, 867

19. HARRISON, P. M. & GREGORY, D. W. [1968], Nature [London] 220, 578

20. PALMER, J. L. & NISONOFF, A. [1964], Biochemistry 3, 863

21. OLIVIERA, B. & LAMM, M. E. [1971], Biochemistry 10, 26

22. KNÜSEL, A. [1971], Pathol. Microbiol. 37, 337

23. WARBURG, O. & CHRISTIAN, W. [1942], Biochem. Z. 310, 384

24. AVRAMEAS, S. & TERNYCK, T. [1969], Immunochemistry $\underline{6}$, 53

25. MILLONIG, G. [1962], 5th Int. Congr. Electron Microscopy, Philadelphia $\underline{2}$, 8

26. LUFT, H. [1961], J. Biochem. Biophys. Cytol. $\underline{9}$, 409

27. GELDERBLOM, H., BAUER, H. & FRANK, H. [1970], J. Gen. Virol. $\underline{7}$, 33

28. GELDERBLOM, H., BAUER, H., BOLOGNESI, D. P. & FRANK, F. [1972], Zbl. Bakteriol. Hyg., Abt. I Orig. A $\underline{220}$, 79

29. GELDERBLOM, H., BAUER, H. & GRAF, T. [1972], Virology $\underline{47}$, 416

30. KURTH, R. & BAUER, H. [1972], Virology $\underline{47}$, 426

31. KURTH, R. & BAUER, H. [1972], Virology $\underline{47}$, 145

32. GELDERBLOM, H. & BAUER, H. [1973], Int. J. Cancer $\underline{11}$, 466

33. SINGER, S. J. & NICOLSON, G. L. [1972], Science $\underline{175}$, 720

34. VALENTINE, R. A. & GREEN, N. M. [1967], J. Molecular Biol. $\underline{27}$, 615

35. PUTNAM, F. W. [1969], Science $\underline{163}$, 633

3.2 In vitro Characterization of Avian Oncornavirus Directed Tumor Antigens

R. Kurth, H. Gelderblom and H. Bauer

The transformation of a normal cell to a malignant state is accompanied by a series of physiological changes. Some of the more
obvious alterations include the change in cell morphology, release from density dependent inhibition of growth, agglutinability
by lectins and appearance ot tumor specific cell surface antigens
(TSSA). In vivo transplantation experiments indicated first that
chemically induced tumors carry individual tumor specific surface
antigens, whereas cells transformed by viruses expose TSSA which
seem to be specific for the group of the transforming virus strain.
No cross-reactions between the TSSA induced by different groups
of oncogenic viruses have thus far been reported (1). However, the
question of strict group-specificity of the induced TSSA is not clar-
ified. Otherwise well studied oncogenic virus groups, e.g., the
avian and murine oncornaviruses, have not yet been compared for
their possible ability to induce cross-reacting tumor antigens.

Origin and role of TSSA in the transformation process is not understood. It is not known whether TSSA are virus-coded or virus-
induced, whether they are newly synthesized, or rearranged or
uncovered macromolecules of the cell membrane. The correlation
between TSSA and embryonic antigens, which can be reexpressed
on transformed cells, also remains to be elucidated.

It was the intention of our work to characterize in vitro the surface
changes accompanying transformation by avian RNA tumor viruses
(ATV). This model is very suitable for basic studies in tumor immunology because of the availability of cloned virus strains with

different biological behaviour and because of the possibility to
study different defined virus–host cell relationships. Among others,
two situations can experimentally be designed which might find
their correlation in human oncogenesis: the activation of latent tumor viruses from normal cells and the transformation of cells
without concomitant virus production.

Material and Methods

Viruses. Avian tumor viruses can be distinguished into avian sarcoma (ASV) and avian leukosis viruses (ALV) according to the a-
bility of ASV only to transform chicken embryo cells (CEC) in culture. The strains can further be classified into five subgroups re-
flecting the antigenicity of their viral envelope antigens (Ve-Ag).
The Ve-Ag also determines host range and interference with other
ATV strains. Table 1 gives examples of virus strains of different
subgroups used in these investigations. RSV (RAV-1) is a pseudo-
type of the BRYAN high titer (BH) strain of ROUS sarcoma virus
(RSV).

Table 1:

Subgroups of avian tumor virus strains used in
these studies.

	Avian Leukosis Viruses[+]	Avian Sarcoma Viruses[++]
Subgroup A	RAV-1, NC-SRV-1	RSV(RAV-1), SRV-1
B	MAV-B, AMV-B	
C		B-77
D	NC-SRV-H	SRV-H

+) unable to transform CEC in vitro
++) able to transform CEC in vitro

It is defective for infectivity, that is, an ALV, here RAV-1, has
to provide an envelope protein in order for the RSV to be infectious.
NC-SRV-1 and NC-SRV-H are mutants obtained after hydroxylamine
treatment of the sarcoma viruses SRV-1 and SRV-H, respectively.
They have lost the capacity of the parental virus strains to transform CEC in vitro (2), but like ALV have retained the capacity to
transform hematopoetic stem cells in vivo (3).

Sensitization. Virus neutralizing chicken sera were obtained after
immunization of the animals with sub-tumorigenic doses of living
ASV or ALV strains (4, 5). Cytotoxic antiserum against tumor specific cell surface antigens (6) was obtained from inbred STU mice
which were immunized at least ten times with cells of a syngeneic
RSV induced mouse tumor.

Cells. Chicken embryo cells derived from L 15 chickens were
used. Cells were either productively infected with ALV or productively infected and transformed with ASV. In addition, ASV
transformed mouse (D4) and hamster (RSH) cells were investigated for their cell surface antigenicity. The properties of the
different cell types are listed in Table 2.

Immunological methods were used to distinguish in vitro between
normal and tumor specific components in the plasma membrane
of ATV transformed chicken, mouse, and hamster cells. Neutralizing chicken sera were used to strain chicken or mammalian
cells by the indirect immunoferritin-hybrid antibody technique (7).
Target cells were first incubated with chicken immune serum and
the bound antibodies were then tagged by hybrid rabbit antibodies.
These antibodies were biochemically prepared to have two specificities: one directed against chicken immunoglobulins, the
other against horse spleen ferritin as the electron dense marker
(see diagram on 3.1, page 134). For indirect immunofluorescence,

Table 2 :

Target cells investigated for ATV-specific cell surface
changes.

Cells	Species	Infected by	Transformation	Virus production	Virus induced antigens
CEC	L-15 chickens	-	-	-	-
CEC	L-15 chickens	different ALV	-	+	Ve-Ag
CEC	L-15 chickens	different ASV	+	+	Ve-Ag, TSSA
MEC	STU-mice	-	-	-	-
D4	STU-mice	SRV-H	+	-	TSSA
HaEC	hamster	-	-	-	-
RSH	hamster	SRV(subgroup not determined)	+	-	TSSA

CEC: chicken embryo cells, MEC: mouse embryo cells,
HaEC: hamster embryo cells.

rabbit immunoglobulins with specificity for chicken antibodies
were conjugated with fluoresceinisothiocyanate. A standard
rabbit antiserum was used to stain chicken antibodies specifically bound to membrane antigens of chicken or mammalian cells
grown on glass coverslips (6). Due to the instability of avian
complement and the inability of chicken immunoglobulins to activate the C'1 component of mammalian complement (8), cellular
instead of humoral cytotoxic microtests were used to detect virus-

induced surface alterations (4, 6). Target cells were seeded out in 10 μl volumes in the 60 wells of Falcon Microplates I, allowing 60 combinations of target and effector cells at various cell ratios. One day later target cells were washed and overlayed with lymphoid effector cells. Either sensitized circulating lymphocytes or sensitized spleen cells were taken as effector cells to investigate their cytotoxic effects after 2 days' incubation with chicken or mammalian target cells. A survival rate for target cells was introduced as follows:

$$\frac{\text{number of surviving target cells incubated with immune lymphocytes}}{\text{number of surviving target cells incubated with normal lymphocytes}} \times 100.$$

Inactivated normal and anti-D4 mouse sera were used in humoral cytotoxic microtests (6). Target cells again were seeded out in Falcon Microplates I one day prior to the exposure to 5 μl normal or antiserum at different dilutions. After 30 min. incubation with serum, 5 μl fresh guinea pig complement were added at a final concentration of 1 : 8. Incubation was continued for another three hours and terminated by washing the wells. Adhering surviving target cells were then stained with GIEMSA and counted. Since no background reduction of target cells by normal mouse serum was observed, cell survival could be taken directly.

Results

First of all, it was necessary to investigate whether infection of CEC by ATV leads to constant cell surface changes. It was found that both, specific ferritin-labeled chicken antibodies and sensitized chicken lymphocytes detect two types of antigens on the surface of CEC infected by ALV or ASV:

1) a subgroup-specific, probably viral envelope antigen on the
   surface of all ATV infected CEC, and
2) tumor specific surface antigens expressed only on ASV transformed chicken cells. These TSSA appear to be group-specific,
   that is, they are cross-reacting on all transformed CEC independent of the subgroup of ASV used for transformation.

Fig. 1 shows the strict subgroup-specific staining of the virus
envelope and the cell surface. Because of this strict correlation,
one can assume that the detected antigen is identical to the Ve-Ag.
It is unclear, whether all Ve-Ag positive areas on the cell membrane represent potential budding sites for viral particles. In the
control Fig. 1c, neither virus particle nor cell membrane are
stained. In Fig. 2, an additional immunological reaction becomes
visible. When antisera prepared against ASV (not ALV) were used,
a group-specific antigen, restricted to transformed cells, appeared.
In the homologous reaction (Fig. 2a), both virus particles and cell
membrane are labeled, whereas in heterologous reactions (Figs.
2b, c) only the cell membranes are stained. We conclude from
this pattern, that anti-ASV sera contain antibodies with specificities for both Ve-Ag on particles and membranes and TSSA on
membranes only.

Essentially identical data were obtained in cellular cytotoxic reactions. As shown in Fig. 3, cytotoxic effects of two different
strengths were exerted on target cells from one embryo infected
by different ATV. Spleen lymphocytes in this example had been
sensitized against NC-SRV-1 and exerted a moderate cytotoxicity
on CEC infected by ALV of the same subgroup (NC-SRV-1, RAV-1).
This reaction is presumably mediated via the Ve-Ag. Again a
second, stronger reaction is evident from the extensive destruction of ASV transformed CEC.

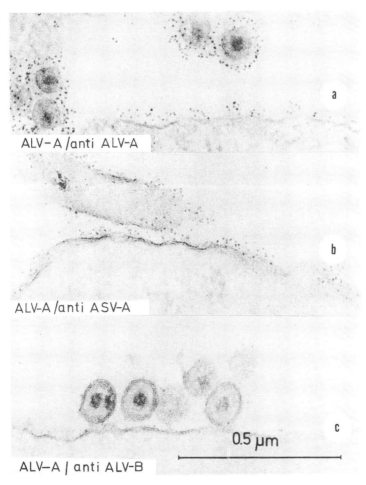

ALV–A /anti ALV-A

a

ALV-A /anti ASV-A

b

ALV–A / anti ALV-B

0.5 µm

c

Fig. 1. Immunoferritin staining of a chicken embryo cell infected
by an avian leukosis virus of subgroup A (ALV-A). Chicken
antisera used for staining were prepared by immunizing
chickens with ALV-A (1a), ASV-A (1b) or ALV-B (1c).

This group-specific effect is thought to be due to the common

expression of cross-reacting TSSA. In those cases where anti-

ALV or anti-ASV lymphocytes were tested on CEC transformed

by an ASV of the same subgroup, the effects are mediated by

both Ve-Ag and TSSA.

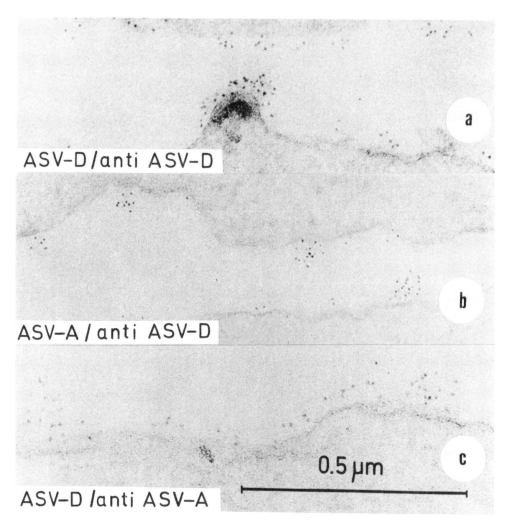

ASV-D/anti ASV-D   a

ASV-A / anti ASV-D   b

0.5 μm   c

ASV-D /anti ASV-A

Fig. 2. Immunoferritin staining of a chicken embryo cell transformed by avian sarcoma viruses of subgroup D (2a, c) or
A (2 b). Chicken antisera used for staining were prepared
by immunizing chickens with ASV-D (2a, b) or ASV-A (2 c).

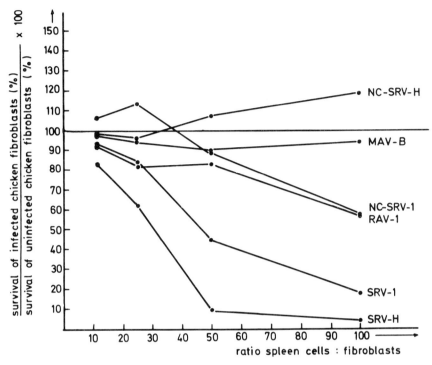

Fig. 3: Cytotoxic effects of chicken spleen lymphocytes sensitized
        against ALV-A (NC-SRV-1). No effect is exerted on target
        cells infected by ALV from a different subgroup (MAV-B,
        NC-SRV-H). A moderate cytotoxicity is seen on CEC in-
        fected by ALV from subgroup A (NC-SRV-1, RAV-1).
        ASV transformed CEC (SRV-1, SRV-H) are always de-
        stroyed to a high extent, irrespective of the ASV-strain
        used for the transformation of target cells.

There is only one discrepancy in the results obtained by the above

two methods. Whereas anti-ALV sera did not detect TSSA in vitro,

anti-ALV spleen cells did. Two reasons could account for this

difference. First, the spleen cells for the microcytotoxicity tests

were taken from hyperimmunized animals, whereas the sera used

for ferritin labeling were derived from animals immunized by a

single injection of virus. Secondly, ALV can transform hemato-

poetic stem cells in vivo, causing, for example, lymphoblastoid leukemias after long latency periods (9). These transformed cells expose TSSA, which, as membrane bound antigens, are preferentially recognized by the host's lymphocytes.

Having established the existence of ATV-specific TSSA on chicken tumor cells, it was of interest to extend these studies to investigate the alterations occurring on mammalian cell surfaces upon transformation by ATV. It had been shown before that the D4 mouse and the RSH hamster cell lines in contrast to transformed CEC do not produce viral particles (10).

For indirect immunofluorescence tests, neutralizing chicken antisera were used (6). Table 2 shows, that the transformed mouse and hamster cells were stained, indicating interspecies cross-reacting TSSA. Fig. 4 is a photomicrograph of stained, transformed D4 and RSH cells. It turned out to be virtually impossible to focus the RSH cells for photography, since they tend to grow in suspension and therefore floated in the glycerol buffer used for mounting the coverslips. Control cultures of MEC and HaEC were not stained.

To substantiate further the existence of interspecies cross-reacting TSSA in ATV induced tumors, inbred STU mice were immunized against syngeneic D4 tumor cells to obtain an antiserum specific for the neoantigens on the tumor cell surface. This antiserum was tested in humoral microcytotoxicity tests (6). Its effects on chicken and mammalian target cells are summarized in Fig. 5. Again only the transformed cells were destroyed, no matter from which of the tested species they were derived. However, whereas D4 and RSH cells were killed to approximately the same extent, transformed CEC always survived at higher antiserum dilutions. This interspecies TSSA was recently also demonstrated on ASV-transformed chicken and mouse cells using the ferritin hybrid antibody technique (11).

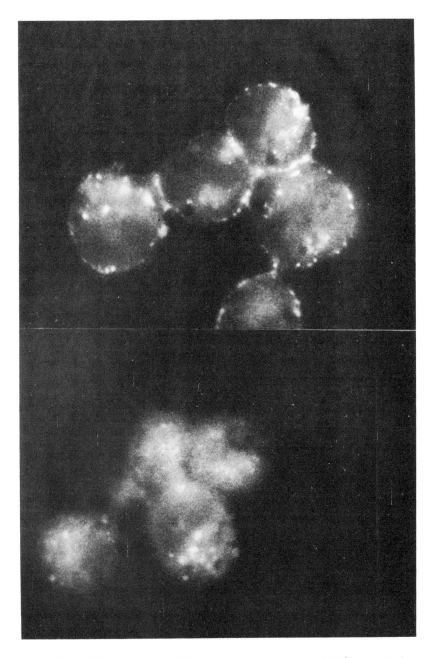

Fig. 4. Positive immunofluorescent reaction of D4 mouse tumor
cells (above) and RSH hamster tumor cells (below).
ASV-neutralizing chicken sera were used, which contain
antibodies recognizing TSSA.

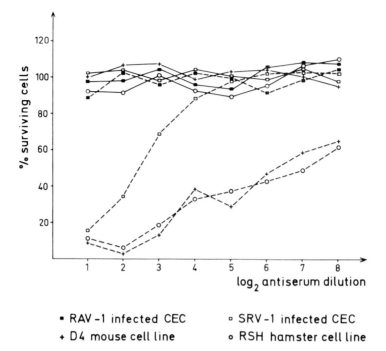

Fig. 5. Effects of normal (solid lines) and anti-D4 (broken lines) mouse serum on chicken and mammalian cells. Only the transformed cell types are destroyed by the antiserum, whereas ALV (RAV-1) infected CEC survive in the presence of anti-D4 serum. Normal serum exerts no cytotoxicity on any of the target cells.

In cellular cytotoxic microtests using anti-D4 sensitized STU mouse spleen cells or ATV-immunized chicken spleen cells, the existence of a cross-reacting TSSA became also evident by the specific destruction of only the ASV-transformed chicken or mouse tumor cells (6). Fig. 6 gives an example of the destruction of D4 tumor cells by chicken spleen cells sensitized against SRV-1 virus.

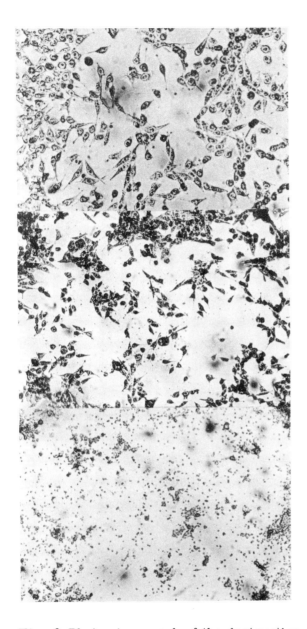

Fig. 6. Photomicrograph of the destructive effects of chicken
spleen cells sensitized against ASV-A (SRV-1 virus) on
ASV-D (SRV-H virus) transformed mouse tumor cells.
Above: mouse cells incubated in medium only.
Middle: ratio effector lymphocytes: tumor target cells 5:1.
Below: ratio effector lymphocytes: tumor target cells 50:1.

Discussion

The use of virus neutralizing chicken sera in an immunoferritin technique and of virus sensitized chicken spleen cells in cellular cytotoxic microtests revealed the existence of two types of antigens on the surface of ATV infected chicken cells. One, a group-specific tumor antigen (TSSA), is restricted to the membrane of ASV transformed chicken cells, while the second, subgroup-specific antigen is also found on ALV infected, nontransformed cells.

Because of the strict correlation between the staining of the virus envelope and the cell surface in the case of the subgroup-specific reaction, one can deduce that the relevant antigen is identical to the viral envelope antigen. This assumption is supported by the finding that the cytotoxic effect of immune spleen cells is re-stricted to those ALV-infected nontransformed CEC, where the infecting virus belonged to the same subgroup as the virus used for immunization. Unlike Ve-Ag, which is distributed without sharp delineations on the surface of infected CEC in large areas of 0,5-2,0 μ, TSSA is present in patches of not more than 200-400 mμ in size 5 . TSSA is either of identical or strongly cross-reacting antigenicity exposed on the plasma membrane of all transformed CEC which we studied, independent from the sub-group of the transforming virus.

Nothing is known about the origin of ATV induced TSSA. Indirect, though not conclusive evidence indicating a viral origin comes from the induction of at least one common antigenic determinant of TSSA on transformed cells from different species. Comparing the cytotoxicity of a given anti-TSSA serum on different target cells (Fig. 5), it becomes obvious that transformed CEC are destroyed to a lesser extent than transformed mammalian cells. This could be due to several reasons. It may be the result of true quantitative differences in the amount of TSSA exposed on the cell surface. Or it may reflect an only partial cross-reactivity of TSSA. That means, some of the antigenic determinants of virally induced TSSA may be shared by all cells transformed by a given virus group, whereas other tumor associated determinants are species-specific. Finally, a more trivial explanation could be derived from the observation that transformed CEC produce high amounts of mucopolysaccharides which cover the outer surface of the cell membrane and may simply prevent the binding of the antibodies to their respective antigenic receptors.

The reexpression of embryonic antigens has been described for animal (12) and human (13) tumors. Again it is not yet known whether these embryonic proteins are newly synthesized or whether they become immunogenic through an uncovering mechanism. Preliminary studies on ATV transformed chicken and mouse cells revealed the existence of at least two types of embryonic antigens: those that are expressed on both normal and transformed cells in culture and in addition those that are tumor associated, becoming reexpressed only after malignant transformation (manuscript in preparation).

Still little is known of the biological function and immunological effects of tumor antigens. As shown by cytotoxicity assays, both Ve-Ag and TSSA can act as transplantation type antigens, with TSSA mediating a much stronger cytotoxic effect than Ve-Ag. In vivo, the basic immunological phenomenon is the constant finding of host lymphocytes sensitized against the autochthonous tumor. Specific antibodies are also demonstrable, which, however, in general are only cytotoxic in those hosts which will eventually overcome their tumor.

A most important immunological factor is the appearance of so-
called "blocking activities" in the serum of hosts with progressively growing tumors (14). These activities prevent in vitro the
killing of tumor target cells by sensitized lymphocytes. It seems
that the blocking effect is due to the existence of either free, non-
cytotoxic antibodies binding to the tumor antigens, to soluble tumor antigen binding to cytotoxic antibody and lymphocytes or to
antigen-antibody complexes with additional free binding sites to
absorb antibodies and antigen (15).

We are now isolating ATV-induced TSSA to characterize them
biochemically. This could be a prerequisite for studies on the
induction of tumor immunity without concomitant induction of
blocking activities. Once this is achieved, vaccination with tumor
antigens becomes practically possible, and several ways are
theoretically open to enhance the comparatively poor immuno-
genicity of tumor antigens to obtain a more potent vaccine. For
example, the introduction of new surface antigens to tumor cells
may lead to a "carrier-effect" resulting in an increased immune
response against the original tumor antigens (16, 17).

Summary

Transformation of chicken and mammalian cells by avian RNA
containing tumor viruses leads to the induction of tumor associated cell surface antigens. In productively infected cells, viral
envelope antigens are also incorporated into the cell plasma
membrane. The interspecies-specificity of the tumor antigens
could be demonstrated by immunoferritin, immunofluorescence,
humoral and cellular cytotoxic techniques. The relevance of
tumor antigens with respect to their potential usefulness in immunotherapy of cancer is briefly discussed.

References

1. HAUGHTON, G. & NASH, D. R. (1969), Progr. Med. Virol. 11, 248

2. GRAF, T. , BAUER, H. , GELDERBLOM, H. & BOLOGNESI, D. P. (1971), Virology 43, 427

3. BIGGS, P. M. , MILNE, B. S. , GRAF, T. & BAUER, H. (1973), J. Gen. Virol. 18 , 399

4. KURTH, R. & BAUER, H. (1972a), Virology 47, 426

5. GELDERBLOM, H. , BAUER, H. & GRAF, T. (1972), Virology 47, 416

6. KURTH, R. & BAUER, H. (1972b), Virology 49, 145

7. GELDERBLOM, H. , This issue.

8. BENSON, H. W. , BRUMFIELD, H. P. & POMEROY, B. S. (1961), J. Immunol. 87, 616

9. BURMESTER, B. R. , FONTES, A. K. , WATERS, N. F. , BRYAN, W. R. & GROUPE, V. (1960), Poultry Sci. 39, 199

10. GELDERBLOM, H. , BAUER, H. & FRANK, H. J. (1970), J. Gen. Virol. 7, 33

11. GELDERBLOM, H. & BAUER, H. (1973), Int. J. Cancer 11, 466

12. TING, C. C. , LAWRIN, D. H. , SHIU, G. & HEBERMAN, R. B. (1972), Proc. Nat. Acad. Sci. USA 69, 1664

13. GOLD, P. & FREEDMAN, S. O. (1965a), J. Exp. Med. 121 , 439

14. HELLSTRÖM, I. , HELLSTRÖM, K. E. , EVANS, C. E. , HEPPNER, G. H. , PIERCE, G. E. & YANG, J. P. S. (1969), Proc. Nat. Acad. Sci. USA 62, 362

15. SJÖGREN, H. O. , HELLSTRÖM, I. , BANSAL, S. C. & HELLSTRÖM, K. E. (1971), Proc. Nat. Acad. Sci. USA 68, 1372

16. MITCHISON, N. A. (1972), in VIth International Symposium on Immunopathology, Grindelwald, p. 52 (ed. Miescher, P. A.) Schwabe-Verlag, Basel

17. KURTH, R. & BAUER, H. (1973), Europ. J. Immunol. 3, 95

3.3 Tumor-Cell Membrane Antigens Related to Blood Group A Substances

O. Prokop, A. Rothe[1] and G. Uhlenbruck[1]

The blood group antigens A, B and H can be detected in normal
human tissues by means of absorption experiments, immunofluorescence or the mixed-cell method. In malignant tumors,
there is often a reduction in or loss of the ABH antigens, due to
the transformation of the cells. This was again demonstrated by
TOMIYAMA [1], who was working under FURUHATA. It was also
demonstrated in 1969 by DAVIDSOHN, KOVARIK and NI [2] in
tissue samples from 82 patients with malignant and benign
changes in the cervical tissue. Their experiments were based
on the mixed-cell method, in which paraffin slices, some of
them more than 10 years old, were loaded with human anti-A and
anti-B sera. Then, where antibodies have been bound, blood
cells with the homologous AB0 group can later be fixed [for
details, see KOVARIK, DAVIDSOHN and STEJSKAL [3]]. Deletion
of the ABH antigens has been described not only in cases of
stomach carcinoma [4-6], but also in carcinomas of the ovary,
cervix of the uterus, lung, and pancreas [6]. In leukemias, even
the erythrocytes loose ABH blood group receptors [review by
UHLENBRUCK and REIFENBERG [7]]. It is also known that
"new" antigen structures appear in suitable tests, in particular
with heterophilic agglutinins [from plants and invertebrates].
"Appear" implies that the structures determined are not necessarily neoantigens, but that known structures which are differ-
ently arranged topographically may appear to be different anti-

1] Supported by a grant from the Landesamt für Forschung, Nordrhein-Westfalen

genically, perhaps because [as can be demonstrated by the action of proteases on ordinary blood cells] a receptor area [a cryptic antigen] which is normally buried has reached the cell surface or now forms it. In some cases the receptor brings its charge with it and thus affects the total charge of the coat [8-11]. Another possibility is that the previously scattered receptors come together in clusters [12].

One antigen of this sort is the "A-like" antigen of certain tumor cells. It is, of course, only one of the tumor antigens in the antigen profile, which includes organ-specific, bacterial, e.g. mycoplasma, fetoprotein antigens, etc.[see ESSERS' review in 1969 [13]]. There has been a great deal of discussion about this antigen, including reference to a possible role in carcinogenesis, since many authors, beginning with AIRD, BENTALL and RO-BERTS in 1953 [14], have indicated that A-carriers are statistically more susceptible to certain malignancies than 0-carriers. Even if the criticism of this work [see PROKOP and UHLEN-BRUCK 1966 [15], which contains many references to WIENER's work] is accepted, there remain, according to VOGEL and HELMBOLD [16], the stomach carcinomas, especially those of the cardia, rectal carcinomas and the salivary gland tumors, in which the relationship to the AB0 system is, as the authors say "definitely indicated".

They mean, to be sure, only "statistically definite". On account of its basis in biological fact, the hypothesis of HELMBOLD [in 16] seems very reasonable. It assumes a selection through differences in the capacity of the host to form antibodies against carcinoma cells.

According to HELMBOLD, an A-group carcinoma cell will also carry an A antigen profile, although this A will be antigenic, due to the changed [with respect to the normal cells] "protein complex" [quotation marks ours]. Let us call it the "A-like" antigen. Antibodies against this antigen will be blocked, however, by the A-substance in the plasma. A biological defense fails, as is not the case in 0-group subjects.

If one wanted to speculate, one could extend HELMBOLD's theory [it is further expounded in VOGEL and HELMBOLD's handbook contribution [16], 1972], with respect to enhancement: Mitosis stimulation in tumor cells by the antibodies provoked by the strong A antigen. The hypothesis could then conceivably be made to agree with the actual observations of A-like structures on tumor cells.

There is at present no uniform definition of "A-like", and it is in any case a phenomenological term. For the time being, it only means that reagents which "otherwise" indicate A receptors also react with cells which are "A-like". There are antibody-like substances with chemically defined specificity which react with A receptors, or part of them, and these are particularly well suited for studies of A-like membrane antigens. A tabular representation of the results obtained with anti-A_{HP} [agglutinin from the protein gland of Helix pomatia] and anti-A_{Db} [from Dolichos biflorus] already provides a certain insight into the problem as it appears today [see tables 1 and 2]. Figure 1 is a summary of the chemical specificity of the reagents which can be used to detect tumor-specific [or relatively specific] antigens, or which are important for determining the chemical specificity.

In fact, we were able to identify positively A antigens on samples of various human tumors, particulary when fluorescence label-ling was used. These results were independently confirmed by other authors during the time of our experiments [BLOOM et al. [17]]. This is an important theoretical advance, but therapeutical-

Table 1:

Possible chemical structure of the A-like antigen on tumor cells as suggested by tests with anti-A_{HP}

Model and comments

a] β-D-GalNac: detected with anti-A_{HP}

Anti-A_{HP} does react with this receptor, but weakly. It was suggested by PROKOP/UHLENBRUCK that this hexosamine could be the tumor receptor, but since anti-A_{CN}, which does not react with the ß-anomer, does react with the tumor antigen, it is unlikely that ß,D-GalNac is the antigen.

Appears when human erythrocytes are treated with RDE [the FRIEDENREICH antigen]. It is present in the substructure of the erythrocyte coat, directly or indirectly blocked by neuraminic acid.

b] α-D-GalNAc: This hexosamine is the main receptor for anti-A_{HP}, but it cannot be the tumor receptor, because the latter is not recognized by anti-A_{Db}.

Occurs on all A-carrying cells, Cad blood group and C Steptococci. There is no experimental model which proposes this hexosamine as a tumor antigen. It does occur in neuraminic acid-free glycoproteins such as submaxillary mucin.

c] α-D-GlcNAc: Anti-A_{HP} reacts with this receptor, which is a probable candidate for the tumor receptor because it, like tumor cells, does not react with the Dolichos reagent.

Dog erythrocytes, which are FORSSMAN-positive but not recognized as "A" by the Dolichos antibody, carry the D-GlcNAc receptor. [This has been determined by inhibition experiments]. They are thus antigenically related to certain tumors [UHLENBRUCK, GIELEN & PARDOE [22]].

d] β-D-GlcNAc: This receptor reacts with anti-A_{HP}, and is reported by HAMMARSTRÖM & KABAT [20,21] to be present on tumor cells, apparently because it also reacts with WGL agglutinin [wheat germ] [UHLENBRUCK, GIELEN & PARDOE [22]].

Substructure element of the carbohydrate chains of many glycoproteins and glycolipids [blood group substances!], often in the form of the disaccharide N-acetyl-lactosamine, from which it can be released by ß-galactosidase [GOTTSCHALK et al. [23]].

Summary: As the A-like tumor receptor: a] is possible,
b] is unlikely,
c] and d] are both likely and much more so than a]

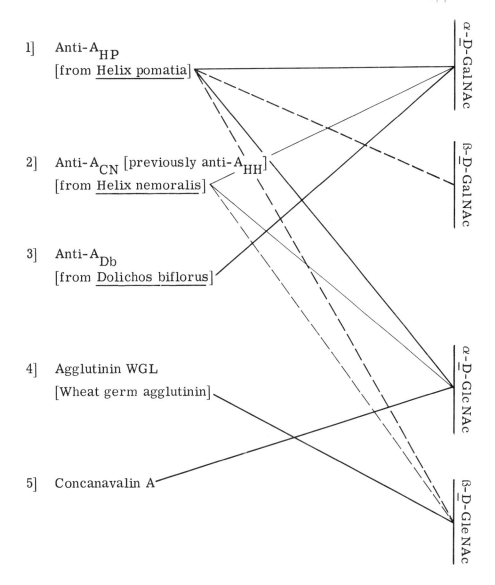

Fig. 1. Hexosamines which could play a role in the A-like
structure. These groups can be detected on the
surfaces of tumor cells or of cells in general with
the listed 5 reagents.

Solid lines, definite specificity, or main specificity

Dashed lines, secondary specificity

Table 2:

Evidence for the A-like structure of tumor cells
[detectable with anti-A_{HP}]

Authors	Material	Results
PROKOP, GRAFFI & SCHNITZLER [1968] [24]	ZAJDELA-hepatoma cells from the rat [ascites tumor cells] Mouse SOV 16 leukemia cells [ascites]	100 to 8000 times more antigen in tumor cells than in normal body cells [erythrocytes].
ARDENNE, KRÜGER, PROKOP, SCHNITZLER [1969] [25]	Mouse EHRLICH ascites cells	
UHLENBRUCK & SEHRBUNDT [1968] [26]	HeLa cells [0] Detroit cells [0]	These are not group A cells, so the tumor cell receptors are tumor-specific.
PROKOP, GRAFFI, HOFFMANN, SCHNITZLER [1968] [27]	Some trypsin-isolated human tumor cells of the B and 0 groups	
PROKOP, UHLENBRUCK, ROTHE, to be published	Baby hamster kidney cells Mouse fibrosarcoma	Transformed cells react strongly with anti-A_{HP} [see also the work of MAKITA & SEYAMA, 1971] [28].

Conclusions:

The tumor cells also react with anti-A_{CN}, but not with the
Dolichos agglutinin. Some of them react with WGL agglutinin.
The probable specificity is thus narrowed to D-GlcNAc. It is
possible, of course, that the A_{HP} and WGL receptors are
simultaneously and independently present, for instance as
receptors on two different carbohydrate chains.

ly [not diagnostically!] our hands are to a certain extent tied. It appears that covering the cell surface with these antibodies [in some cases also those from external sources] obscures the "true" tumor antigens or makes them sterically inaccessible, so that the specific cellular immunity, which is much more important for rejection of tumors and transplants, is unable to operate. The tumors thus grow faster and better in the presence of the antibodies. We have therefore gone a more roundabout way and have tried to mark specifically the T-lymphocytes, which are so important for the defense against tumors. Using the anti-A-like agglutinin, we were able to identify both the tumor cell antigens and the anti-tumor T-type cells. Furthermore, of the neuraminidase-treated lymphocytes, which react strongly with anti-A_{HP} [7,18], only the T-lymphocytes are involved, and not, as we previously assumed, all of them. The solution of this problem with respect to the immunocompetent cells, which are so important to tumor immunology, and their reaction with the agglutinin anti-A_{HP} will have far-reaching clinical and scientific consequences [19].

The discovery of A-like tumor antigens on certain kinds of tumor cells has led us to consider therapeutic or diagnostic applications. To be sure, binding of the antibody to the tumor cell membrane does not necessarily imply a therapeutic effect. If anti-A_{HP} is injected into the ascites of animals with A_{HP}-positive ascites tumors, it has no effect on the tumor or the survival time of the animal. There is no indication that anti-A_{HP} could have a mitogenic effect, because it does not stimulate lymphocytes as PHA [phytohemagglutinin] does [18]. The protectin anti-A_{HP} is also incapable of cytolysing the cells, due to its inability to bind complement. However, advantage has been taken of its binding capacity by using anti-A_{HP} as a carrier for cell poisons. Anti-A_{HP} could not be bound to NOL [nitrogen mustard gas], but it did bind to DOC [sodium deoxycholate], and the combination was successfully tested in the trypan blue test with EMAC [EHRLICH mouse ascites tumor cells] [25]. It is important for a possible application to humans that intravenous application of anti-A_{HP} to monkeys was well tolerated [29], although a molecular weight of 100 000 is not inconsiderable. It is, however, a moderately strong antigen for rabbits, apparently with a certain antigenic relationship to pigs. Two new papers have shown that it is actually able to react with certain tumor cells in vitro and in vivo. ARDENNE and CHAPLAIN [30] treated thin slices of human ovarial, cervix and vaginal tumor tissue with ^{125}I-labeled anti-A_{HP} and measured the degree of binding in a gamma counter. The tumors belonged to blood groups B and 0. The result was that, especially in the interzone tumor hosts, the young tumor cells bound the antibodies. The authors noticed that not only the especially invasive cells [limit of detection 10^6 cells], but also in one case, bronchial lymph node metastases carried the A-like receptors.

FINCK and VOGLER [31] applied for the first time anti-A_{HP} which had been labeled with ^{131}I by the chloramine method. The preparation had an activity of 300 μCi and was tolerated without any problems. It was used with 0 and B patients, and it was possible to identify moderately well a bronchial carcinoma. The labeled antibody was also detected in the liver [it is a glyco-protein, after all], and was quickly excreted through the kidneys.

Binding of the antibody to liver cells in vitro was not demonstrated, so that it must be assumed, with certain reservations, that anti-A_{HP} was either metabolized in the living liver, or that the preparations used were not pure and contained labeled ballast substances.

On reviewing the experiments which have been published to date, one can see that a new field for extensive studies has been opened. If it actually turns out that D-GlcNAc plays a role on the surface of certain tumor cells, then the way is clear for a diagnostically useful tumor antigen. That this hexosamine is in fact involved in the tumor receptors of certain defined tumors is suggested by the experiments of SHIER [32], who has tested a chemical vaccine against tumor progress. He has coupled D-GlcNAc to polyasparaginic acid and bovine albumin, and has found that mice immunized with it rejected 5 times as many tumor cells as non-immunized animals.

Other work in this direction, referred to elsewhere [UHLEN-BRUCK and REIFENBERG [7]], is concerned with the immunization against neuraminidase-treated leukemia cells. We now know that there is a strong A-like antigen on these enzyme-treated cells which can be detected with anti-A_{HP} [UHLEN-BRUCK, VAITH and SCHUMACHER [18]], and which appears to be very important.

In conclusion, we can say that there are quite characteristic changes in the antigen mosaic and topographical architecture of tumor cell membranes which can be detected with heterophilic agglutinins, but not with the classical immunological methods.

References
1. TOMIYAMA, K. [1957], Acta Orimin. Med. Leg. Jap. 23/3, 2
2. DAVIDSOHN, I., KOVARIK, St. & NI, L. Y. [1968], Arch. Pathol. 87, 306

3. KOVARIK,St.,DAVIDSOHN,I. & STEJSKAL,R.[1968],Arch. Pathol. 86,12

4. HÄKKINEN,I.[1970],J.Nat.Cancer Inst. 44,1183

5. SHEAHAN,D.G.,STANISLAV,A.,HOROWITZ,A. & ZAMCHECK,N.[1972],Digest.Dis. 16,961

6. DAVIDSOHN,I.,NI,L.Y. & STEJSKAL,R.[1971],Cancer Res. 31,1244

7. UHLENBRUCK,G. & REIFENBERG,U.[1972],Einige Anmerkungen zur Antigenität von Leukämiezellen, in Leukämie [eds.Gross,R. und Van de Loo,J.]Springer-Verlag, Berlin-Heidelberg - New York

8. UHLENBRUCK,G. & REIFENBERG,U.[1971],Med.Klin. [Munich] 66, 1435

9. PROKOP,O. & UHLENBRUCK,G.[1969],Med.Welt 46, 2515

10. BURGER,M.M.[1971],Cell surfaces in neoplastic transformation, in Current Topics in Cellular Regulation, vol. 3,p.135, Acad.Press, New York

11. BEN-BASSAT,H.,INBAR,M. & SACHS,L.[1971], J.Membrane Biol. 6, 183

12. SINGER,S.J. & NICOLSON,G.L.[1972],Science 175,720

13. ESSERS,U.[1969],Deut.Ärztebl. 38, 2589

14. AIRD,I.,BENTALL,H.H. & ROBERTS,J.A.F.[1953], Brit.Med.J. I, 799

15. PROKOP,O. & UHLENBRUCK,G.[1966], Die menschlichen Blut- und Serumgruppen, 2.Aufl., Thieme-Verlag,Leipzig

16. VOGEL,F. & HELMBOLD,W.[1972],Blutgruppen-Populationsgenetik und Statistik, in Humangenetik [ed.Becker,P. E.]Thieme-Verlag, Stuttgart

17. BLOOM,K.[1973] J.Cancer 12, 21

18. UHLENBRUCK,G.,VAITH,P. & SCHUMACHER,K.[1972], Naturwissenschaften 59,220

19. UHLENBRUCK,G.,WERNET,P. & SCHUMACHER,K. [1973],Klin.Wochenschr. 51, 1210

20. HAMMARSTRÖM,St. & KABAT,E.A.[1969],Biochemistry 8, 2696

21. HAMMASTRÖM,St. & KABAT,E.A.[1971],Biochemistry
10,1684

22. UHLENBRUCK,G.,GIELEN,W. & PARDOE,G.I.[1970],
Z.Krebsforsch. 74,171

23. GOTTSCHALK,A.,SCHAUER,H. & UHLENBRUCK,G.[1971],
Z.Physiol.Chem. 352, 117

24. PROKOP,O.,GRAFFI,A. & SCHNITZLER,St.[1968],Acta
Biol.Med.Germ. 20/K, 9

25. ARDENNE von, M.,KRÜGER,W.,PROKOP,O. & SCHNITZ-
LER,St.[1969],Deut.Gesundheitsw. 24/13, 588

26. UHLENBRUCK,G. & SEHRBUNDT,H.[1968],Klin.Wochenschr.
46,905

27. PROKOP,O.,GRAFFI,A.,HOFFMANN,F. & SCHNITZLER,
St.[1968],Deut.Gesundheitsw. 41,1926

28. MAKITA,A. & SEYAMA,Y.[1971],Biochim.Biophys.Acta
241,403

29. ARDENNE von,M.,PROKOP,O.,FLEISCHER,J.,SCHNITZ-
LER,St.,KRÜGER,W.,LAPIN,B.A.,ANNENKOW,H.A.,
ASSANOW,N.S. & KOLODIN,V.I.[1970],Deut.Gesund-
heitsw. 18,817

30. ARDENNE von,M. & CHAPLAIN,R.A.[1972],Naturwissen-
schaften 59/6, 278

31. FINCK,W. & VOGLER,H.[1972], Radiobiol. Radiotherap.
2, 267

32. SHIER,W.T.[1971],Proc.Nat.Acad.Sci.USA 68, 2078

3.4 Erythrocytic ABH-Receptors in Leukemia – An Immunofluorescence Study [1]

K. Fischer and A. Poschmann

In the past several years, various authors have reported (1-6) changes in the ABH-properties of erythrocytes from leukemia or tumor patients. When the blood was typed it was noticed that only a part of the erythrocytes agglutinated with anti-A, anti-B or anti-H. Two reaction types are to be emphasized: In one type, A or B receptors are replaced by an increased number of H receptors, while in the other, a reduction in the number of A or B receptors is not accompanied by an increase in the number of H receptors. The abnormal development of the ABH system reported in the literature was discovered by agglutination reactions and absorption and elution experiments. A change in the ABH receptors of a single erythrocyte cannot be detected with these techniques. In the Abteilung für Immunpathologie, we have had many years of experience with our own immunofluorescence technique, with which it is possible to detect the erythrocyte receptors on a single erythrocyte (blood smear) (7-11).

The principle of this technique is presented in Figure 1. Unfixed blood smears are incubated with the test reagent (globulin). After washing, a fluorescein-labeled antiglobulin is used to make the test reagent bound to the receptors (e.g. anti-A to A) visible. For these experiments, we purified agglutinins from humans, animals and plants and immunized rabbits with them. The antiglobulins so obtained were marked with fluorescein isothiocyanate.

1) Supported by a grant from the Deutsche Forschungsgemeinschaft

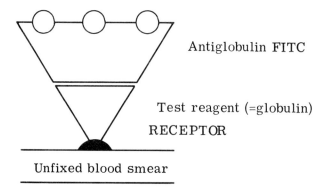

Fig. 1.   Indirect immunofluorescence technique for the
detection of erythrocyte receptors.

Together with the Abteilung für Gerinnungsforschung und Onkologie (Direktor: Prof. Dr. G. LANDBECK) of our clinic, we have
been able to examine the blood of 2 children with chronic myeloic
leukemia. A detailed description will follow in another place(12).
Here we wish to limit ourselves to the immunological results.

An unusually high quantity of HbF-containing erythrocytes (94.6%)
was found in the blood of the first, five-year old child by the
acid elution technique (13). The child's blood belonged to group
A_2, but the agglutination of his erythrocytes with the reagents
anti-A_{hu} (human origin), anti-A_{La} (phythemagglutinin from
Laburnum alpinum) and anti-BH_{Ee} (phythemagglutinin from
Evonymus europaea) was, in comparison to the reaction of his
father's A_2 erythrocytes, noticeably weak and incomplete. The
mother belonged to blood group 0. The titers are shown in
Table 1.

In order to determine the distribution of these receptors on the
individual erythrocytes, we carried out immunofluorescence
experiments with IgG-anti-A and anti-BH_{Ee}.

Table 1:

Reaction of the A and H receptors of a child with chronic myeloic leukemia with agglutinins of various specificities

Patient Chr. born 10. 6. 67	Angela "A_2"	Father A_2
HbF cells	94. 6 %	2. 9 %
Anti-A_{hu}	4 part.	32
Anti-H_{La}	4 part.	8
Anti-BH_{Ee}	16 part.	16

In Figure 2a, only a few erythrocytes with various amounts of A receptors are visible, in contrast to the normal A_2 develop- ment in the father's blood (2 b) . The picture in the blood of new- borns of blood group A_2 is the same as in the child with chronic myeloic leukemia. In the infants, the individual erythrocytes display widely varying amounts of A receptors, which is an indication that the A property is not yet completely mature. The BH_{Ee} receptors were similarly reduced. We can designate this kind of change in the receptors as the fetal type, since not only the high concentration of HbF, but also the visibility of the A and BH_{Ee} receptors on the erythrocytes correspond to the physiological conditions of the fetal period.

Following these first experiments, we were able to expand considerably the immunofluorescent determination of the recep- tors, which are arranged in a mosaic-like pattern around the genetic A and B receptors. In addition to various phythemag- glutinins with anti-H specificity, we used "protectins" from the protein glands of various species of snails (14-16) which deline- ate the mosaic of the A partial receptors. Since some of the

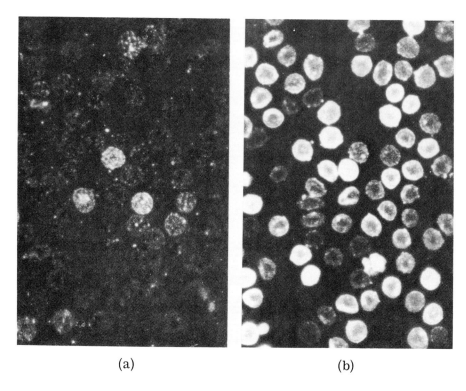

(a)   (b)

Fig. 2 a and b.   Determination of A receptors from an A_2 child
                    with chronic myeloic leukemia (a) with IgG-
                    anti-A. Comparison with the A_2 father (b).
                    Blue-light fluorescence. Ortholux fluorescence
                    apparatus (Leitz): mercury high-pressure
                    lamp CS 100 W (Philips), illumination fluores-
                    cence, exciting light filter BG 12 (1. 5 mm),
                    interference filter S 470, interference divider
                    plate 495 nm (lens turret No. 3), blocking filter
                    K 530, objective F 1, oil 54/0.95 (Leitz) , auto-
                    matic microscope camera Orthomat (Leitz) ,
                    Ilford H P 4 (29 DIN) film

receptors which can be detected with these reagents are also
present as cryptic antigens, which can only be detected after the
removal of acetylneuraminic acid, we did additional experiments
using neuraminidase from Vibrio cholerae (receptors destroying
enzyme = RDE from Behringwerke).

The second child, 7 years old, has a chronic, myelomonocytic leukemia. In the blood group type test, there was partial agglutination with anti-A and anti-A_1. Later tests revealed 30% A_1 and 70% of the erythrocytes which did not react with anti-A or anti-B, and thus behaved in this respect like 0 erythrocytes. Therefore we called this fraction the "0" fraction to distinguish it from the A_1 fraction. Figure 3a shows two sharply differentiated erythrocyte populations revealed by indirect immunofluorescence using IgG-anti A. Figure 3b shows the immunofluorescence of mature A_1 erythrocytes as they are normally found after the first year of life.

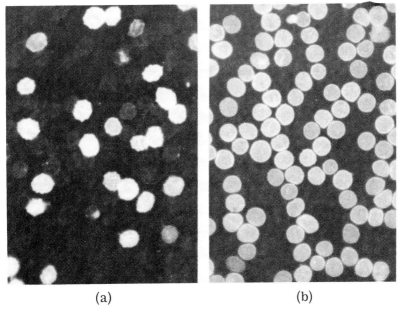

(a)   (b)

Fig. 3 a and b.   Two erythrocyte populations: in chronic myelomonocytic leukemia (a), and normal A_1 erythrocytes (b), for comparison. Immunofluorescence with IgG-anti-A.

To determine whether the child belongs to the A or 0 blood group, we examined the saliva. The child excreted A antigens. For further tests, we separated the two populations by differential agglutination with human anti-A. In this process, we eluted the anti-A from the A_1 fraction by adding A blood group substance. Thereafter we examined the individual fractions, using various reagents for the A and H complexes, with the agglutination technique, and in part with the indirect immunofluorescence technique.

Table 2:
    Reaction pattern of the A complex and H complex with the blood of a child with chronic myelomonocytic leukemia. Agglutination reaction in NaCl medium.

Patient P. L. born 15. 2. 65	Whole blood	A_1 fract.	"0" fraction native	"0" fraction RDE	A_1	Controls 0	Controls 0_{RDE}
Anti-A_{hu}	256 p	64	–	–	128	–	–
Anti-A_{Db}	4 p	16	–	–	32	–	–
Anti-A_{HP}	2000 p	2000	–	8000	512	–	2000
Anti-A_{HA}	128 p	128	8	256	128	–	256
Anti-A_{CH}	256 p	512	–	4 p	256	–	–
Anti-A_{CN}	2000 p	2000	–	16 p	1000	–	–
Anti-H_{La}	–	–	–	256	–	32	512
Anti-H_{Ue}	8 p	–	8	128	–	16	128
Anti-BH_{Ee}	8 p	–	64	8000	–	128	4000

As Table 2 shows, the whole blood reacts partially with all the test reagents. The isolated A_1 fraction behaves as normal A_1 blood. The "0" fraction, however, does not behave as normal 0 blood; it does not react with anti-H_{La} (from Laburnum alpurnum), although the anti-H reagents from Ulex europaea (anti-H_{Ue}) and Evonymus europaea (anti-BH_{Ee}) show a normal reaction. If we were to designate this fraction as 0 blood, there would be a defect in the formation of the receptor H_{La}. The tests with the anti-A reagents also revealed a reaction pattern which corresponds neither to normal A_1 blood nor to normal 0 blood: anti A_{HA} (from Helix aspersa) reacts positively, although more weakly than with the A_1 control. However, in contrast to the normal A_1 control, the native "0" fraction reacts negatively in the agglutination tests with the reagents anti-A_{Db} (from Dolichos biflorus), anti-A_{HP} (from Helix pomatia), anti-A_{CH} (from Cepaea hortensis) and anti-A_{CN} (from Cepaea nemoralis). Furthermore, the receptors A_{CH} and A_{CN} are present in the "0" fraction of cryptic antigens, which are revealed by treatment with neuraminidase. These receptors are not found in normal 0 blood, even after enzymatic cleavage of the acetylneuraminic acid. The reaction with anti-A_{CH} and anti-A_{CN} involves only a part of the erythrocytes of the "0" fraction. Immunofluorescence tests (Fig. 4) showed that only a few erythrocytes fluoresce with anti-A_{CH} and anti-A_{CN}. The fraction of the erythrocytes agglutinated by these reagents is larger, which suggests an uneven distribution of the A_{CH} and A_{CN} receptors.

Figure 5 summarizes the results from the second child. In contrast to normal A_1 blood, the "0" fraction lacks the receptors A_{hu}, A_{Db} and A_{HP}; the receptor A_{HA} is present in a weak form, and the receptors A_{CH} and A_{CN} are present only as cryptic antigens. In contrast to normal 0 blood, the receptor H_{La} is missing. Thus this fraction has lost most of the receptors of the A complex, but additional receptors for H_{Ue} and BH_{Ee} are present, which cannot be detected in the normal A_1 fraction with the agglutination technique used.

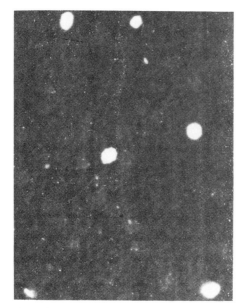

Fig. 4.　Immunofluorescence of the A_{CN} receptors in the
neuraminidase-treated "0" fraction.

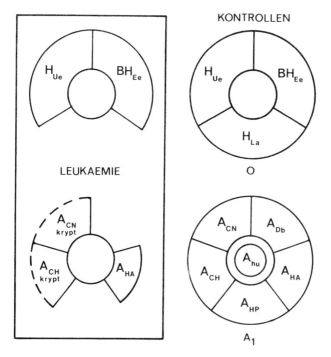

Fig. 5.　Loss of receptors and additional receptors in chronic
myelomonocytic leukemia

In contrast to the fetal type of ABH receptor change, in which partial loss of receptors occurs on all erythrocytes, there are in this second type two distinct erythrocyte populations. The A_1 fraction reacts normally, but the "0" type must be considered defective. A similar situation is found in blood chimeras, where A_1 stem cells have been transferred to an 0 fetus, and for this reason, we propose to call this pattern of receptor changes the chimera type. The fetal and chimera types have partial hemagglutination in common and can only be distinguished by the immunofluorescence technique.

Summary

Changes in the erythrocyte ABH receptors in chronic myeloic leukemia are reported. An immunofluorescence technique developed by one of us makes it possible to determine the erythrocyte receptors on individual cells (blood smear technique). The results obtained with this technique reveal two characteristic types of changes in erythrocyte receptors, 1) the fetal type, with various levels of receptor loss from all the erythrocytes, and 2) the chimeric type, with two sharply distinguished erythrocyte populations, one with a normal receptor mosaic and the other with a loss of receptors. Partial hemagglutination occurs in both types. The different types can be distinguished only by the immunofluorescence technique.

References

1. VAN LOGHEM, J. J., DORFMEIER, H. & VAN DER HART, M. (1957), Vox Sang. 2, 16

2. STRATTON, F., RENTON, P. H. & HANCOCK, J. A. (1958), Nature (London) 181, 62

3. GOLD, E. R., TOVEY, G. H., BENNEY, W. E. & LEWIS, F. J. W. (1959), Nature (London) 183, 892

4. MICHAELS, L. & McNAMARA, E. (1962), Lancet 1962, 512

5. DUCOS, J., RUFFIE, J., MARTY, Y., SALLES-MOURLAN, A. M. & COLOMBIES, P. (1964), Nature (London) 203, 432

6. BARTOVA, A. (1965), Zur Frage des Vorkommens der in der ABO-Antigenität abweichenden Erythrozyten bei Hämoblastosen und malignen Tumoren, Proc. 10th Congr. Int. Soc. Blood Transf., Stockholm 1964, p. 330 (1965), Karger-Verlag, Basel - New York

7. FISCHER, K. & STEGE, N. (1967), Vox Sang. 12, 145

8. FISCHER, K. & POSCHMANN, A. (1969), Zum Nachweis erythrozytärer Rezeptoren mit der Immunfluoreszenztechnik, Vortr., 1. Tagg. Ges. Immunol., Freiburg/Breisgau, Oktober 1969

9. FISCHER, K., POSCHMANN, A. & OSTER, H. (1971), Monatschr. Kinderheilk. 119, 2

10. POSCHMANN, A., FISCHER, K., REUTHER, K. & MYLLYLÄ, G. (1974), Persistent mixed field polyagglutinability. An immunofluorescence study in genetically abnormal red cells, Vox Sang. (in press)

11. FISCHER, K., POSCHMANN, A. & WINTERSTEIN, K. -H. (1972), Darstellung des Rh-Faktors D an mütterlichen und kindlichen Erythrozyten mit der Immunfluoreszenztechnik, Vortr. 5. Deut. Kongr. Perinat. Med., Berlin, November 1972

12. POSCHMANN, A., FISCHER, K., KURME, A., WINKLER, K. & LANDBECK, G., Chronische, myeloische Leukämie (juveniler Typ) mit Veränderung der ABH-Rezeptoren. Immunfluoreszenzuntersuchungen (in preparation)

13. KLEIHAUER, E. & BETKE, K. (1960), Internist 1, 292

14. PROKOP, O., RACKWITZ, A. & SCHLESINGER, D. (1965), South African J. Forens. Med. 12, 108

15. PROKOP, O., SCHLESINGER, D. & RACKWITZ, A. (1965), Z. Immunitätsforsch. Exp. Klin. Immunol. 129, 402

16. GOLD, E. R. & THOMPSON, T. E. (1969), Vox Sang. 16, 119

3.5 Immunological Aspects of Placental Choriocarcioma

E. Robinson

Choriocarcinoma of the placenta is known to originate from the fetal chorion and represents a disorder of the trophoblastic growth. This tumor is unique in that it is derived from the tissue of the patient and her husband. It may develop after full term delivery, miscarriage or hydatidiform mole. In recent years there has been a considerable interest in the immunological aspects of this tumor. The survival and growth of the trophoblastic tumor, which is believed to carry potent antigenic determinants which are not shared by the mother in an immunologically adverse maternal environment, has led to some interesting questions and speculations. If the tumors are antigenic, why does the immune response not eliminate them? Why is the fetus, which is antigenic, only rejected after 9 months?

It was suggested [1] that the prognosis of choriocarcinoma may be related to the degree of histocompatibility between the tumor and its host. Good prognosis is indicated in a patient with choriocarcinoma when the mating can not produce zygotes histocompatible with the mother and especially if antibodies active against HL-A antigen of her husband are found.

The purpose of our study is to examine the relationship between the patient and her husband, in order to see whether close histocompatibility between them exists, this being responsible for the tumor growth, or whether acquired maternal tolerance or desensitization induced by foreign antigens of the fetus is responsible.

Experiments

Fourteen patients with choriocarcinoma were studied. Full thickness skin grafts from their husbands were transplanted to their right forearm and split skin graft from random donor for comparison was transplanted to their left forearm. The grafts were followed up from the fifth post-operative day by two different observers.

The leucocytic isoantigens were studied following a previously described technique [2].

In the patient with active tumor the survival of husband's skin graft was significantly prolonged 4 - 10 weeks. In two patients the grafts were excised and examined histologically. The examination confirmed the survival of the graft. In 2 patients cured of their disease by chemotherapy, the husband's skin graft underwent accelerated rejection [white graft]. The skin grafts from normal donors were rejected in all cases within 10-15 days.

The result of leucocyte antigen studies shows that there is no compatibility between husband and wife [4].

Discussion

Choriocarcinoma is a rare tumor in Western countries and frequent in the Far East. Its incidence in Western countries is 1 : 13,850 live births, in Israel 1 : 15,000 live births and in Taiwan 1 : 496 live births [5]. Therefore, in order to reach conclusions a pooling of material from various countries is necessary.

It was found that foreign donor homograft was rejected on time, meaning that the immune mechanism of the patient reacted normally toward it. Only the reaction to the husband's skin graft was impaired. MATHÉ et al.[6], BAGSHAWE [7] and LI [8] have confirmed our findings of delayed husband homograft rejection in women with advanced choriocarcinoma and accelerated rejection in cured patients. This, together with leucocyte antigen studies supports the theory that there is no histocompatibility between the patients and their husbands.

Various authors have studied the blood groups in patients with choriocarcinoma. Some investigators found a normal ABO distribution [9]. Others found less patients in group 0 [10,11]. It was also seen that patients with AB group tended to have a rapid growing tumor. The highest risk was found in women of group A married to a male of group 0, whereas women of group A married to males of group A showed the lowest risk. The spontaneous regression of trophoblast after evacuation of hydatidiform mole happens most commonly in women mated to males of their own ABO phenotype [12,13,14].

The histocompatibility antigens have been shown to be at least partially identical to the leucocyte or tissue antigens. Therefore, various authors thought it of importance to study these antigens in patients and their husbands. Van ROOD found that some patients had one allele in common with their husbands and others none [15].

JABOUBKOVÁ et al.[16], AMIEL et al.[17] and LAWLER et al. [14] and the author [4] found that the frequency of HL-A2 antigen was similar in patients and the general population. The patients were also not more compatible with their husbands than a comparable group of normal couples [14] [see table 1].

Table 1 Immunological and serological findings in chorio
carcinoma

Blood Groups

Author	Year	Results
SCHMIDT and HERTZ	1961	Normal ABO distribution.
SCOTT	1962	Less patients in group 0.
BAGSHAWE	1970	AB group tended to have rapid growing, resistant to chemo-therapy.
BAGSHAWE	1970	Women of group A $_{0-highest\ risk}$ married to male group$_{A-lowest\ risk}$

Leucocyte Antigens

Author	Year	Results
Van ROOD	1968	Some patients had one allele in common with their husband, others none.
JAKOUBKOVÁ et al.	1970	Incompatibility in HL-A2 antigen.
AMIEL	1970	Frequency of HL-A2 was similar in patients and general population.
ROBINSON	1967	Patients were not more compatible
LAWLER	1971	with husbands than a comparable group of normal couples.

Leucocyte and Platelets Antibodies

Author	Year	Results
DONIACH et al.	1958	Found antibodies.
DAUSSET	1959	2 cases with antibodies.
MATHÉ et al.	1964	3 out of 5 had antibodies.
JAKOUBKOVÁ et al.	1970	40% of 32 patients had antibodies.
SHULMAN	1964	Found antibodies.
RUDOLPH and THOMAS	1971	44 patients.
ROBINSON et al.	1967	No antibodies.

Antigen Compatibility and survival

	No. Patients	No. Antigens in common	Condition of Patients
MOGENSEN et al.	16	0	1 death
	29	1 ore more	5 deaths
MILLER	2	0	2 localized disease
	11	1	8 generalized disease
	2	2	2 generalized disease

The chance of survival was greater among the patients who were most
incompatible with their husbands.

Suggestions for Incompatibility

LAWLER et al.	Cho. occurs in the presence of HL-A incompatibility
RUDOLPH and THOMAS	
Van de PUTE et al. and others	Cytotoxic antibodies have been found in cured and dead patients.
LEWIS et al.	High percentage of transformed cells in
HALBRECHT et al.	mixed lymphocyte culture.
ROBINSON et al.	No HL-A compatibility. No leucoagglutinins.

Patients Reaction to the Tumor

1. The incidence of malignant change in molar pregnancy increases with age.
2. Different behaviour and reaction to treatment of chorio-carcinoma in women and men.
3. Few authentic cases of spontaneous regression have been reported.
4. The improvement obtained by immunotherapy.

MOGENSEN and KISSMEYER-NIELSEN reported that there is a correlation between the number of antigens in common between the husband and the patient and the survival. The chance of survival was greater among the patients who were most incompatible with their husbands [18,19].

The possibility of having specific antibodies against the spouse antigen was investigated by various authors. There were authors who reported that they had patients who had leucoagglutinins [6, 20,21] and others not [22,23,3]. It has been investigated whether those patients who had leucoagglutinins would show an accelerated rejection of primary skin graft from their spouse. Accelerated rejection did not occur. The cause of this could be explained by tolerance. The fact in favour of this is that no compatibility between the patient and her husband was found [1,18,19]. LAWLER et al [14], RUDOLPH and THOMAS [22] have shown the presence of choriocarcinoma in patients with HL-A incompatibility. There was also no correlation between the presence of cytotoxic antibodies and the survival. Antibodies were found in both patients who were cured and those who died [13] [see table 1].

Mixed lymphocyte culture is a vitro immunological reaction which depends upon immunogenetic differences or related to the HL-A locus [24]. In mixed lymphocytic culture between patients and their husbands a high percentage of transformed cells has been found indicating incompatibility [25,26].

There is various evidence of an immune reaction against the choriocarcinoma:
1. Histological examination of the tumor shows in a variable degree the presence of clusters of mononuclear cells in the tissue adjacent to the choriocarcinomatous masses. The presence of a well marked cellular reaction is associated with better prognosis [27].
2. The incidence of malignant change in molar pregnancy increases with age [28]. In advanced age immunodepression is stronger and the incidence of malignant neoplasm is higher.
3. Few authentic cases of spontaneous regression of choriocarcinoma were reported [29, 30].
4. There is a different behaviour and reaction to treatment in women and men. The placental choriocarcinoma can be cured by chemotherapy and that of the male not [31]. Choriocarcinoma of the male and female heterotransplanted separately to each cheek pouch of the hamster reacted similarly to the treatment with methotrexate [32]. The possible explanation is that also in the patient both tumors react equally to methotrexate. But in the woman, by reducing the tumor mass, methotrexate succeeds also in breaking the tolerance to the tumor. At this point, the

mechanism of the woman recognizes the foreigness of the tumor and is able to destroy the tumor cells left. In the non placental choriocarcinoma the tumor cells are not foreign and therefore the results are not as good.

DONIACH et al.[20] tried to immunize a female patient immediately after ablation of the tumor by dermal injection of spouse leucocytes and the application of husband skin graft. The course of illness did not change. CINADER [33] immunized one of his patients with husband spermatoids with some effect. Other authors used husband lymphocytes, also with some effect [34, 35, 36].

One of our patients who did not react to chemotherapy was treated with husband's leucocytes once. As the immunological studies showed no compatibility we continued the treatment with FREUND's adjuvant in order to stimulate antibody production of the husband's antigens already present in the woman. After this treatment the abdominal mass disappeared and the pulmonary metastases decreases in size and number. However, the patient died suddenly. At autopsy the cause of death was found to be an intestinal perforation at a place where some nests of tumor mass were found [37]. Surgery with chemotherapy should be considered as the principal methods of treatment. Immunotherapy should be given only to patients resistant to this treatment.

The tumor cannot be rejected by the patient although we have found that there is no compatibility between the husband and the wife. The surface of the trophoblast contains paternal antigens but certain configuration in the cell periphery appears to mask the antigenic site [38]. This masking is not absolute and the woman becomes immunized against the husband's antigens. BARDAWIL and TOY [39] suggested that the survival of the choriocarcinoma in a patient may be the result of prior conditioning of the maternal stroma by normal trophoblast. The shower of syncytial trophoblast that becomes deported to the lungs during normal pregnancy may serve a similar purpose by enhancing the growth of a later chorionic neoplasm. This enhancement has been described by KALISS as a factor in the growth of experimental tumor [40].

Summary

Leucocyte antigen and leucoagglutinin studies, ABO blood groups, skin graft transplantation and the results of immunotherapy, favor the theory that immune tolerance is responsible for the husband's prolonged skin graft and may be the cause why the placental choriocarcinoma is not rejected.

Choriocarcinoma can be cured by surgery and/or chemotherapy, such as methotrexate, vinblastine or actinomycin. The drugs have a cytotoxic affect directly on tumor cells. Reducing the number of cells most probably breaks the tolerance, enabling the immune system of the patient to destroy the remaining tumor cells.

In resistant cases to chemotherapy, immunotherapy by itself should be tried.

References

1. MOGENSEN, B. & KISSMEYER-NIELSEN, F. [1969], Danish Med. Bull. 16, 243

2. GILBOA, N. & NELKEN, D. [1961], Nature [London] 192, 466

3. ROBINSON, E., SHULMAN, S., BEN HUR, N., ZUCKERMAN, H. & NEUMAN, Z. [1963], Lancet I, 300

4. ROBINSON, E., BEN HUR, N., ZUCKERMAN, H. & NEUMAN, Z. [1967], Cancer Res. 217, 1202

5. MATELON,M.,PAZ,B.,MODAN,M. & MODAN,M.[1972], Amer.J.Obstet.Gynec. 112,101

6. MATHÉ ,G., DAUSSET,J.,HERVET,E.,AMIEL,L., COLOMBANI,J. & BRULE,G.[1964],J.Nat.Cancer Inst.33,194

7. BAGSHAWE,K.D.[1970],International Cancer Congress Houston,p.206

8. LI,M.C.[1971],Ann.Int.Med. 74,102

9. SCHMITT,P.J. & HERTZ,R.[1961],Amer.J.Obstet. Gynec. 82,651

10. SCOTT,J.[1962],Amer.J.Obstet.Gynec. 83,185

11. LLEWELLYN-JONES,D. [1955],J.Obstet.Gynec.Brit. Common W. 72,242

12. BAGSHAWE,K.D., RAWLINS,G.,PIKE,M.C. & LAWLER, S.D.[1971],Lancet I, 553

13. BAGSHAWE,K.D. & LAWLER,S.D.[1971] Lancet II,1152

14. LAWLER,S.D.,KLOUDA,P.T. & BAGSHAWE,K.D.[1971], Lancet II, 834

15. Van ROOD,J.J.,Van LEEUWEN,A.,SCHIPPERS,A. & BALNER,H. [1968],Cancer Res. 28, 1415

16. JAKOUBKOVÁ,J.,MAJSKY,A.,IVASKOVÁ,E.,ZAVADIL, M. & SNAJD,V. [1970],Neoplasma 17, 223

17. AMIEL,J.L. & LEBOVICI,S. [1970],Rev.Europ.Études, Clin.Biol. 15, 191

18. MOGENSEN,B. & KISSMEYER-NIELSEN, F. [1971], Transplantation Proc. 3, 1267

19. MILLER,R.W. [1971],Transplantation Proc. 3, 1273

20. DONIACH,I.,CROOKSTON,J.H. & COPE,T.I.[1958],J. Obstet.Gynec.Brit.Comm. 65, 553

21. DAUSSET,J. [1959], Sang. 30,634

22. RUDOLPH,R.H. & THOMAS,E.D.[1971],Lancet I,408

23. SHULMAN,N.R.,MARDER,V.J.,HILLER,M.C. & COLLIER,E.M.[1964],Progress in Haematology p.222, Grune and Stratton,N.Y.,London

24. LANG,J.M.,OBERLING,F.,TONGIO,M.M.,MAYER,S. & WAITZ,R. [1972], Lancet I, 1261

25. HALBRECHT, J. & KOLMOS, L. [1968], J. Obstet. Gynec. 31, 173

26. LEWIS, J., WHANG, J., NAGEL, B., OPPENHEIM, J. J. & PERRY, S. [1966], Amer. J. Obstet. Gynec. 96, 287

27. ELSTON, C. W. [1969], J. Path. 97, 261

28. CHAN, D. P. C. [1967], UICC Monograph Serie Vol. 3, 37

29. BARDAWIL , W. A., HERTIG, T. A. & VELARDO, J. T. [1957], Obstet. Gynec. 10, 614

30. EVERSON, T. C. & COLE, W. H. [1956], Ann. Surg. 144, 366

31. HERTZ, R. [1959], Ann. New York Acad. Sci. 80, 262

32. PIERCE, G. B., MIDGLEY, A. R. Jr. & VERNEY, E. L. [1962], Cancer Res. 22, 563

33. CINADER, B., HAYLEY, M. A., RIDER, W. D. & WARWICK, O. H. [1961], Canad. Med. Ass. 84, 306

34. HACKET, G. & BEECH, M. [1961], Brit. Med. J. , 1123

35. SCOTT, J. S. [1962], Brit. Med. J. I, 638

36. JAKOUBKOVÁ, J., KOLDOVSKÝ, P., BEK, V., MAJSKY, A., SCHNEID, V. & VOPATOVÁ, M. [1965], Neoplasma 12, 531

37. ROBINSON, E. & RATZKOWSKI, E. [1965], Gynaecologia 160, 87

38. CURRIE, G. A., van DOORNINCK, W. & BAGSHAWE, K. D. [1968], Nature [London] 219, 191

39. BARDAWILL, W. A. & TOY, B. L. [1959], Ann. N. Y. Acad. Sci. 80, 197

40. KALISS, N. [1962], Ann. N. Y. Acad. Sci. 101, 64

4 Methods for Detection of Non Tumor Antigens and Fetal Proteins

4.1 Non Tumor Antigens in Human Tumors

P. Koldovský, J. Weinstein and H. Lischner

Introduction

The search for specific anti-tumor immunity has been carried
on for almost one hundred years. From the diagnostic and
therapeutic point of view, the most important seems to be the
tumor specific, transplantation antigen [1]. This antigen is known
to elicit the immune reaction, which in turn can influence tumor
growth. TSTA has been found in many experimental tumors and
there is growing evidence that it exists in most, if not all, human
malignancies [2]. It is necessary however to understand the
functions of all cell membrane antigens which the tumor cell
shares with its tissue of origin in order to isolate the function
of TSTA.

The benign cell membrane contains many antigens when the cell
is transformed; new antigens such as TSTA are formed, some
antigens persist, some disappear, and some may disappear and
reappear [CEA]. This study deals with two types of antigens
which may be present after malignant transformation, the organ-
specific antigens and embryo-specific antigens in the brain, kidney
and in intestinal tumors of human origin.

Material and Methods

Target cells: Cells were prepared from normal and malignant
tissue by mincing and placing tissue fragments into growth medium BME 10% FCaS. The bottles were incubated for 48 hours
in a CO_2 incubator at $37^{O}C$. The cells were incubated and
utilized in the 3rd or 4th passage.

Anti-sera: 1. Human sera were obtained from healthy donors,
cancer patients at various stages of the disease, and pregnant
women. The sera were inactivated at $50^{\circ}C$ for 30 min. and used
immediately or stored at $-20^{\circ}C$.

2. Anti-sera were prepared in inbred guinea pigs [strain # 13]
by immunization with whole cells or fresh tissue mixed with
FREUND's adjuvant. The guinea pigs received 4-6 injections and
were bled by cardiac puncture one week after the last injection.
The sera were inactivated and stored at $-20^{\circ}C$.

Absorption of sera: Prior to absorption serum was diluted 1:2 or
1:4 and exposed to washed, packet cells, equal to 1/5 of the
serum volume.

Preparation of white blood cells: White blood cells were obtained
from heparinized whole blood by plasma gel sedimentation or the
direct removal of the buffy coat.

Tests: Cell mediated immunity was measured in microplates II
[Falcon] by the microcytotoxic method described by TAKASUGI
and KLEIN [3]. Fresh guinea pig serum was used as a source of
complement. This serum was pretested and shown not to influence the growth of cells used in these experiments.

The binding of inactivated serum [human or guinea pig] to the
target cells was measured by indirect radioimmunoassay of
HARDEN and McKHANN [4]. About 10^{-3} target cells were placed
in growth medium and seeded on the flat bottom of microplate
wells and incubated at $37^{\circ}C$ for 24-48 hours under CO_2. Following incubation the medium was removed and 0.05 ml of the test
serum was added to each well and the plates were then incubated
for 30 min. under CO_2 at $37^{\circ}C$. The test serum was removed
and the wells were washed with PBS containing 10% fetal calf

serum. I^{125} labeled anti-human or guinea pig gammaglobulin [5] was added to the wells and the plates incubated at $37^{O}C$ under CO_2 for 30 min. The wells were again washed with phosphate buffered saline containing 10% fetal calf serum. The plastic microtiter plates were then cut so that each well could be measured separately for radioactivity.

Results

A] Appearance of embryo antigen of the transplantation type in colon adenocarcinoma: Several types of carcinoembryonic antigens have been previously described [6]. Cells were prepared from 4 adenocarcinomas of the digestive tract, and skin from the same patients, as well as skin, lung, kidney, intestine and brain from 3 months old human embryos. The cytotoxic activity of sera from cancer patients, pregnant women, and controls was tested an these cells utilizing the micro-cytotoxicity test with fresh guinea pig serum diluted 1:10 as a source of complement. Sera from 7 patients with digestive tract adenocarcinoma, 7 pregnant women, and 3 patients with unrelated cancers were used to test cytotoxic activity to target cells derived from an adenocarcinoma [BT13] and another unrelated tumor [BT17]. The results shown in Table 1 indicate that sera from adenocarcinoma patients and some pregnant women show cytotoxic activity against cells derived from the adenocarcinoma. No cytotoxic activity was detected in the control sera or in positive sera against control [skin derived] cells.

The data in Table 2 compare the activity of 4 sera, 2 from adenocarcinoma patients [13,2] one from a pregnant woman [9] and one from an unrelated cancer patient [25 - brain tumor] against cells derived from 3 adenocarcinomas [BT13,CA2,CA4], skin cells derived from the donor of tumor BT13, cells from an unrelated tumor [BT17] and cells from embryonic intestine show sensitivity to the sera obtained either from the adenocarcinoma patients or the pregnant woman.

Table 1:

Activity of human sera against adenocarcinoma cells in vitro

Source of serum and serum number	Adenocarcinoma cells	
	BT13	BT 17
Adenocarcinoma patients		
1	16	<2
2, 3, 12	8	NT
11, 13	8	<2
14	4	NT
Pregnant women		
4, 7	2	<2
5, 8	2	NT
6, 10	< 2	NT
9	4	<2
Carcinomatic patients		
18, 25, 44	< 2	

Table 2:

Activity of various human sera against cells from
various patients

Cell	Serum no.			
	13	2	9	25
BT13	8	8	2	<2
C13	<2	<2	<2	<2
BT17	<2	<2	<2	<2
CA2	8	4	2	<2
CA4	16	4	4	<2

Antisera were prepared in guinea pigs to the adenocarcinoma
[BT13] and the embryonic intestine [El]. Prior to and after extensive absorption with white blood cells pooled from whole blood
samples from 30 healthy donors and various normal human cell
lines, the sera were tested against embryonic tissues [intestine,
lung] adenocarcinoma derived cells [BT13,CA2,CA4] and skin
obtained from one adenocarcinoma patient. The results are
summarized in Table 3. Antiserum against the BT13 cells, absorbed with normal cells react only with adenocarcinoma and
embryo intestine. A similar reaction was obtained with antiserum prepared to embryonic intestine [El] against adenocarcinoma and embryo intestine cells. This reactivity from anti-
BT13 sera can be specifically absorbed by both: BT13 and El
cells [and vice versa]. These results indicate that both the
embryonic intestine cells and colon adenocarcinoma cells contain a common cell membrane associated antigen.

Table 3:

Activity of GP antisera against human embryo and tumor cells

Cells	Antisera					
	Non-absorbed		Absorbed with normal tissue		Absorbed with embryo or tumor tissue	
	Anti-BT13	Anti-EI	Anti-BT13	Anti-EI	Anti-BT13	Anti-EI
Embryo intestine	256	256	16	16	<2	<2
Embryo lung	256	512	<2	<2	<2	<2
BT13	512	256	32	16	<2	<2
C13	256	512	<2	<2	<2	<2
CA2	NT	NT	16	8	NT	NT
CA4	NT	NT	16	8	NT	NT

B] <u>Organ specific antigens in human tumors</u>: Tumor cells, brain and skin, were obtained from the same patients. For comparative experiments brain and kidney cells were derived from rabbit, sheep and mouse. Sera were prepared in inbred guinea pigs against normal human brain and syngeneic guinea pig brain. The antihuman brain sera were absorbed with various normal human tissue until no reaction to the normal human lines could be detected. The guinea pig serum against guinea pig brain was antibrain specific without absorption. The anti-human brain serum, following absorption with normal human cells, was specifically cytotoxic to cells derived from human brain tumor and corresponding brain cells. The results shown in Table 4 indicate that the serum was cytotoxic against human brain cells [B25, B11, B9], brain tumor cells [BT12, BT25, BT28], and sheep and mouse brain cells but not against human skin [N25, N11], human diploid cells [W138], SV_{40} transformed human cells [2RA], mouse kidney cells or other types of human tumor cells [BT13, BT11].

The activity of the anti-guinea pig brain antiserum was tested against cells derived from 2 brain tumor patients using the indirect I^{125} binding technique. The cells were prepared from brain tumors [BT27, BT28], brain [B27, B28], and from skin [N27, N28]. As a control, sera were obtained prior to immunization of the guinea pig. The results are represented in Figure 1. It is evident that only the brain tumor and brain cells bind antiserum. No binding was detected with normal skin cells or by normal guinea pig serum.

In similar experiments cells derived from 2 WILM's tumors [WT11, WT12] were studied. Anti-kidney antiserum was prepared by immunizing inbred guinea pigs with whole syngeneic kidney tissue.

Table 4:

Cytotoxic activity of guinea pig anti-human brain serum
absorbed with pooled human leukocytes and various normal
human cell lines

Cells	Titer	Cells	Titer	Cells	Titer
B25	8	BT13	<2	Sheep brain	32
N25	<2	BT12	32	Mouse brain	16
B11	64	BT17	<2	Mouse kidney	<2
N11	<2	BT25	16	2RA	<2
B9	16	BZ28	16	WI38	<2

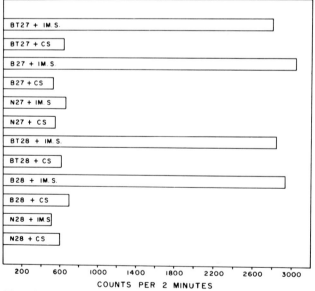

Fig.1.

The binding capacity of the guinea pig and kidney sera was again measured using the indirect I^{125}labeled antibody technique. The results are illustrated in Figure 2.

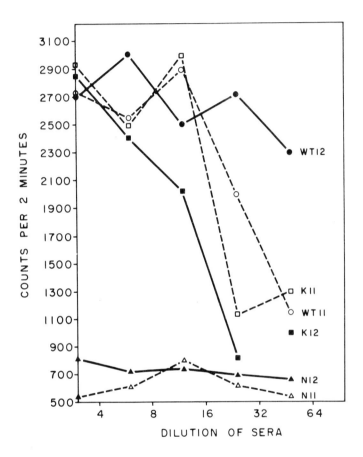

Fig. 2.

The data indicate that the background binding is not dependent
on the titer of the guinea pig sera. All kidney and kidney tumor
cells, however, at a dilution of 1:2 show a 4-6 fold increase in
the number of counts. At a 1:16 dilution the number of counts
were twice that of the control. The data also show that the
WILM's tumor cell [WT12] may contain more of the organ specific
antigen than the normal kidney [K12].

Discussion

The presence of TSTA in many animal tumors has been well
documented [1] and the evidence for the presence of similar antigens in human tumors is also quite convincing. One interesting
difference can be noticed however in animal tumor systems. The
TSTA is specific for a given oncogenic virus [this being common for e.g. all polyoma virus induced tumors regardless of
strain and species of origin] or specific for a given individual
tumor when the tumor is induced by other means [7]. The results
of in vitro experiments with cells derived from human tumors
indicate the presence of common antigens for a given group of
tumors [2]. Conclusions may be drawn from animal experiments
which indicate that a given group of human tumors may be induced
by the same type oncogenic virus or that other antigens can be
responsible for the cross reaction? Thus far no virus has been
linked directly as the cause of human tumors. In the experiments
presented here two antigens were followed which can cause cross
reactions. The first antigen may be the CEA of the transplantation
type, which can be demonstrated in cells derived from human
digestive tract cancers using human or heterologous sera [8].
The second antigen may be organ specific which can be present
in the cells after malignant transformation [8]. It has been
previously demonstrated using heterologous antisera that organ

specific antigens are present in astrocytoma [brain specific] and kidney tumor [kidney specific] [9]. The presence of additional antigens [embryonic, tumor, organ], however, not shared by counterpart tissues cannot be excluded by these experiments.

It must be pointed out, however, that the search for non-tumor specific antigens in human tumors is almost as important as the search for the tumor-specific antigens. The more knowledge one obtains dealing with the antigenic changes at the cell surface the better one may understand malignant transformation and immunology of tumor growth. Such search is as well very important from practical point of view. In the case of organ-specific antigens to prevent unwanted autoimmune reactions. The cancer-embryoantigen of transplantation type has large immunotherapeutical potentialities.

References

1. KOLDOVSKÝ, P. [1969], Tumor-Specific Transplantation Antigen, Springer-Verlag, Berlin - Heidelberg - New York

2. HELLSTRÖM, I. [1971], Int. J. Cancer 7, 1

3. TAKASUGI, M. & KLEIN, E. [1971], The methodology of microassay for cell-mediated immunity, in In vitro Methods in Cell-Mediated Immunity [ed. Bloom, B.] P. Glade AP.

4. HARDEN, F.H. & McKHANN, C.F. [1968], J. Nat. Cancer Inst. 40, 231

5. HUNTER, W.M. & GREENWOOD, F.C. [1962], Nature [London] 194, 495

6. KOLDOVSKÝ, P., SAWICKI, V. & KOPROWSKI, H. [1972], Cross reactivity between SV_{40} transformed cell surface antigen and early embryo antigen, in Cellular Antigens [ed. Nowotny, A.] Springer-Verlag, Berlin - Heidelberg - New York

7. SJÖGREN, H.O. [1964], Progr. Exp. Tumor Res. 6, 289

8. KOLDOVSKÝ, P. & WEINSTEIN, J. [1972], Presence of organ specific antigen and embryo antigen in human tumors, in Conference on Cell-Mediated Immunity in Human Tumors [eds. Herbermann, R. and Levine, P.] J. Nat. Cancer Inst., Monograph

9. WALLACE, A.C. & NAIRN, R.C. [1972], Cancer 29, 977

4.2 Detection of Alpha-1 Fetoprotein in Human Serum

J. B. Smith and R. A. Knight

Introduction

Fetus-specific serum proteins, usually alpha-1 globulins, have now been demonstrated to occur in all animal species tested [1,2,3]. Alpha-1 fetoprotein [AFP], the most extensively studied of these species-specific serum proteins, generally reaches peak concentrations in fetal serum during the early part of the second trimester of gestation and subsequently disappears from the serum, or falls to very low levels, in the perinatal period [3].

The recurrence of high concentrations of AFP in adult serum was first noted by ABELEV [4] in mice bearing primary hepatomas. Later, TATARINOV [5] noted an analogous phenomenon in humans with hepatocellular carcinoma, and this observation was quickly confirmed by other workers [6,7,8,9,10] who recorded that AFP was present in serum from 40-90% of adult patients with primary hepatoma.

The occurrence of increased levels of AFP in adult serum is not specific for the presence of primary hepatoma, although AFP can be used as a screening test in geographic areas where hepatoma is common [10]. High levels of this protein are also found in germinal cell tumors of the testis and ovary [6,11,12,13], occasional patients with other neoplasms [14,15,16,17], Indian childhood cirrhosis [18] and in partial biliary atresia [SMITH, J.B. - previously unpublished].

The introduction of more sensitive AFP assays has resulted in a further lessening of diagnostic specificity and the demonstration of small elevations of AFP in serum from patients recovering from viral hepatitis [13,17,19,20], cirrhosis of the liver [20] after partial hepatectomy [21], in patients with ataxia telangiectasia [22] and during normal pregnancy [13,23,24,25]. Increased amounts of AFP have also been noted to occur in amniotic fluid from women bearing fetuses with anencephaly or spina bifida [26]. Finally, studies using radioimmunoassay indicate that normal adult human serum may contain up to 2 nanograms/ml of AFP [27].

Table 1 indicates the lower limits of sensitivity for several methods of AFP detection and thus indicates some of the limitations imposed by the methods used. It is clear that easily reproducible, highly sensitive and quantitative assays for AFP are needed. Radioimmunoassay meets these requirements and has been used in a number of recent studies [22,24,25,27,28,29].

In this paper we review production of anti-AFP antiserum, purification of AFP, several established AFP assay methods and report on our experience with the development of a radioimmunoassay.

Materials and Methods

Production of anti-AFP antiserum: Antiserum to AFP may be produced by hyperimmunization of adult rabbits with AFP, usually in the form of fetal serum or amniotic fluid, emulsified in FREUND's complete adjuvant [7]. A reasonable immunization schedule which we have found to yield high titer antiserum consists of an initial intramuscular injection of the AFP-adjuvant mixture followed in 6 weeks by a booster intramuscular injection of the same material.

Table 1 :

Occurrence of alpha fetoprotein in adult human serum and methods of detection. Numbers in parentheses indicate approximate lower limits of sensitivity of various assays

I.   Double diffusion [2 micrograms/ml]

Hepatocellular carcinoma   [5,6,7,8,9,10]
Embryonal carcinoma, testis [6,11,12,13]
Choriocarcinoma, ovary [17]
Yolk sac carcinoma +
Occasional other non-hepatic tumors [14,15,16,17]
Hepatitis ++ [17]
Partial biliary atresia +

II.   Immunoradioautography, sandwich counterelectro-phoresis aggregate hemagglutination [100 nanograms/ml]

Acute viral hepatitis [13,17,19]
Partial hepatectomy [21]
Pregnancy   [13,17,23]

III. Radioimmunoassay [< 10 nanograms/ml]

Ataxia telangiectasia [22]
Hepatic cirrhosis [20]
Normal human serum [24,28]

+ SMITH, J. B. - previously unpublished

++ Two cases reported by ABELEV [17]

Three weeks after the first booster injection an intravenous injection of AFP without adjuvant is given and the rabbit is bled 14 days later. Unless the AFP used as the immunogen is highly purified a polyvalent antiserum is produced and absorption of the antiserum is necessary in order to obtain mono-specificity. Usually, this absorption can be effected by mixing the polyvalent rabbit antiserum with pooled normal human serum in a ratio of 1:2 and incubating this mixture at room temperature for 1-2 hours and at $5^{o}C$ for 16-24 hours. After incubation the precipitate formed is removed by centrifugation. It is then preferable to treat the antiserum with an equal volume of saturated ammonium sulfate, centrifuge, resuspend the precipitate in distilled water and dialyse against 0.9% saline to obtain a crude gamma globulin fraction.

Anti-AFP antiserum thus prepared should form a single precipitin line when reacted with fetal serum in double diffusion and this reaction should form a line of immunologic identity with a known positive sample [Fig. 1].

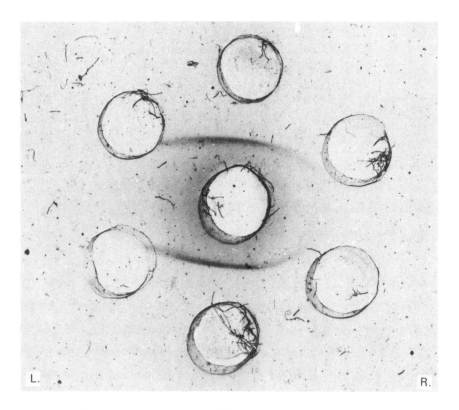

Fig. 1. Double diffusion in 1.0% agarose. Mono-specific anti-AFP antiserum in the central well is reacting with strong precipitin lines with positive AFP control sera in the upper and lower wells. The wells on the right side each contain serum with about 2.0 micrograms AFP/ml, and the two wells on the left contain normal adult serum.

Purification of AFP: Purification of AFP can be accomplished according to the following scheme. Human fetal serum, amniotic fluid or other source of AFP, is mixed with an equal volume of saturated ammonium sulfate and the precipitate formed is separated by centrifugation. This precipitate is then washed once with 50% saturated ammonium sulfate, re-centrifuged, and dissolved in distilled water. After dialysis against 0.9% saline for 24-48 hours this material is concentrated by pressure dialysis and subsequently subjected to passages through two different anti-adult human serum antibody columns and a mono-specific anti-AFP column. The purified AFP is eluted from the final column with glycine-HCl buffer at pH 2.4. Antibody columns are prepared according to the method of AXEN and PORATH [30] which utilizes cyanogen bromide to co-valently link antibody to Sepharose 2-B [Pharmacia, Uppsala, Sweden]. Columns thus prepared remove normal adult serum components from the AFP preparation and the resultant material, again after concentration, should react with monospecific anti-AFP antiserum but not with a variety of anti-whole human serum antisera. In our hands, 4-5 ml fetal serum yields 1-2 mgm purified AFP.

Double diffusion: Glass plates with a 2 mm thick coating of 1.0% agar or agarose in veronal buffer, pH 8.2-8.6 are satisfactory for either double diffusion or electrophoretic methods. Diffusion patterns vary, but we have had success with six 2 mm diameter wells placed around a central well of the same size, such that the outer wells are evenly spaced 2.5 mm from the center well [Fig.1]. Anti-AFP antiserum is placed in the central well and reference positive samples are placed in two of the peripheral wells such that each of the four test sera are in wells bordering on a known positive. Therefore it is not necessary to re-test for immunologic identity should one of the test samples react with the antiserum. Diffusion is allowed to occur for 12-24 hours, after which time plates are scrutinized for precipitin lines. Generally, it is not necessary to stain plates, but if staining is desirable plates should be washed in 0.9% saline for 24-48 hours, dried under wet filter paper, and stained with a general protein stain such as amido black or azocarmine.

Counter-electrophoresis [CEP]: This rapid method is more sensitive than double diffusion but is somewhat more wasteful of antiserum. Two mm wells are cut 4 mm apart in diffusion plates as described above. Anti-AFP antiserum is placed in the well nearest the anode and serum to be tested is placed in the opposite cathodal well. Electrophoresis is carried out for about 40 min. at 10-12 mA, 50-100 V, and at the end of this time a line of precipitation can be seen between the two wells if AFP is present [Fig.2]. It is mandatory to have at least one known reference positive AFP sample in each electrophoresis run. Immunologic identity can be tested by arranging the wells in a triangular fashion [Fig.3] with the anodal well being at the apex and the two test wells forming the base.

Sandwich counter-electrophoresis [SCEP]: This method [13,19], while detecting very low concentrations of AFP is somewhat cumbersome and requires careful interpretation. CEP is done initially for 40 min. using monospecific anti-AFP antiserum in the anodal well. The antibody well is then cleared of fluid by suction and antiserum to rabbit immunoglobulin, purified by ammonium sulfate precipitation and fractionation on DEAE cellulose [Pharmacia, Uppsala, Sweden] in 0.02 M phosphate buffer at pH 7.2, is then placed in the anodal well. Electrophoresis is carried out for an additional 30 min. after which time precipitin bands are sought. Occasionally an overnight wash in 0.9% saline helps to define lines of precipitation. Identity can be tested as with

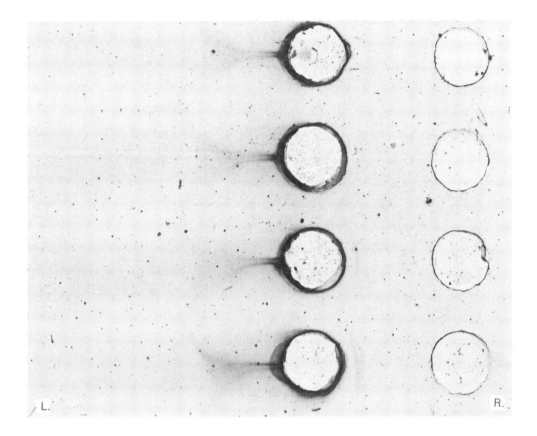

Fig. 2. Counter electrophoresis [CEP] with anti-AFP antiserum placed in the anodal [left side] wells and test samples in the cathodal wells [right side]. After electrophoresis for 40 min. precipitin bands occur between the two lower sets of wells, indicating presence of AFP. The lower precipitin band appears to be split and this is seen occasionally when high concentrations of AFP are present.

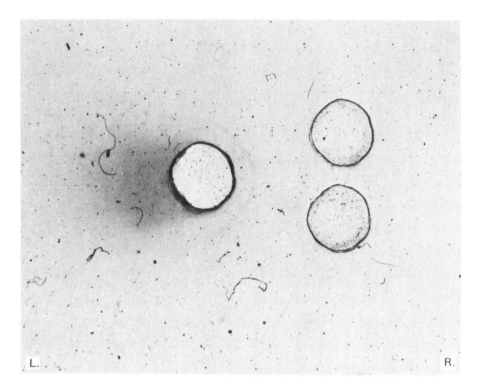

Fig. 3. Identity testing in counter electrophoresis or SCEP. The antiserum to AFP is, again, in the anodal [left sided] well and the test serum is in the upper well on the right. A known AFP + serum is in the lower right well and after 40 min. electrophoresis a precipitin band forms near the antibody well. A line of immunologic identity is formed between the test and known positive samples.

CEP. Presumably, precipitin lines which form in the gel but which are not visible after the initial CEP are intensified by the sandwich antibody. Non-specific precipitation is not a problem as the sandwich immunoglobulin is travelling in a wave behind the rabbit immunoglobulin.

Indirect immunoradioautography [IR]: This method, devised by ABELEV [17] is based on the increased sensitivity of double diffusion when both antiserum and antigen are in very low concentration. The precipitin lines formed at these dilutions are invisible however and are detected by the later addition of ^{125}I-labeled anti-gamma globulin antibodies and subsequent autoradiography.

Radioimmunoassay [RIA]: RUOSLAHTI and SEPPÄLÄ [27,28]and others [25,29] have reported that AFP levels below 10 nanograms/ml can be detected by RIA. To prepare the labeled protein we use a modification of the chloramine-T method [31]. 200 μCi [125]I [Radiochemical Center, Amersham, England], 50 μg of purified AFP and 50 μg chloramine-T are mixed in a total reaction volume of 100 μl and the reaction is stopped after 20-30 sec. by the addition of 100 μg sodium metabisulfite. Either gel-filtration on Sephadex G-75 [Pharmacia, Uppsala, Sweden] or anion exchange using Dowex AG1-X2 [BioRad,Richmond,California] is used to separate labeled protein from unreacted nuclide. Trichloroacetic acid will precipitate 88-96% of protein labeled in this fashion and, after concentration, labelled AFP reacts in double diffusion and forms a line of identity with "cold" AFP when specific antiserum is used. To obtain an antibody dilution curve, 100 μl of labelled AFP, diluted in veronal buffered saline to give about 2000 gamma emissions per minute [Wallac gamma sample counter, Turku, Finland], is added to 100 μl volumes of serial dilutions of antiserum and incubated one hour at room temperature and overnight at 4°C. Baseline gamma emissions are counted and 100 μl of sheep anti-rabbit gamma globulin diluted 1:2 and 100 μl of a 1:40 dilution of normal rabbit serum are then added to separate antibody bound from unbound label. After a further one hour incubation at 37°C the mixture is centrifuged for 15 min. at 2500 rpm, the supernatant is removed by suction and the precipitate is counted. Fig. 4 shows a curve obtained by this method.

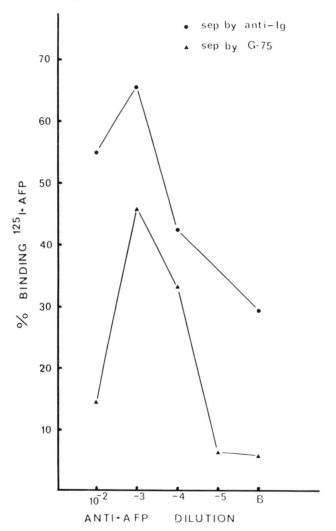

Fig. 4. Antibody dilution curve [see text] showing that 66% of radio-labeled AFP can be precipitated by anti-AFP antiserum in a dilution of 1:10.000 when a sandwich anti-rabbit gamma globulin is used to separate bound from unbound label [upper curve] and that 47% of ^{125}I AFP can be separated at the same antibody dilution by passing the reaction mixture through a 5 cm G-75 solumn [lower curve].

This reaction of labeled AFP with anti-AFP antiserum can be inhibited by "cold" AFP but not by human serum albumin. We have not yet fully investigated the sensitivity of the method.

We have tried various methods of separating bound AFP from unreacted AFP and, using an anti-immunoglobulin, one can bind up to 66% of labeled protein. Ammonium sulfate precipitation of immune complexes is not satisfactory as this causes precipitation of unbound AFP as well and preliminary results using 47.5-55% saturation with ethanol indicate only 10-15% net binding.

Discussion

The number of conditions in which increased amounts of AFP are demonstrable in serum is continually expanding. The detection of more than 1-2 μg/ml of AFP in adult human serum remains highly suggestive of the presence of either hepatoma or germinal cell neoplasia. At concentrations less than 1 μg/ml these tumors may still be present but the finding must then be interpreted with the knowledge that a number of other conditions, chiefly those associated with liver parenchymal hyperplasia, may also be associated with the finding of increased AFP levels in the serum.

It is probable that future studies on the occurrence of AFP in various disease states will continue to be useful in the study of carcinogenesis and regenerative liver states, and it is also probable that AFP determination will continue to be a useful adjunct to the diagnosis of hepatoma and germinal cell neoplasma. The use of AFP determination in following the course of patients after hepatectomy and liver transplantation [32] and during the treatment of neoplasia [33] should also prove to be a useful clinical application.

Acknowledgements

This work was supported in part by grant PF 822 from the American Cancer Society, Inc. [JBS], and by the Medical Research Council of Great Britain [RAK],

References

1. PEDERSON, K. O. [1944], Nature [London] 154, 575

2. BERGSTRAND, C. P. & CZAR, B. [1956], Scand. J. Clin. Lab. Invest. 8, 174

3. GITLIN, D. & BOESMAN, M. [1967], Comp. Biochem. Physiol. 21, 327

4. ABELEV, G. I. [1963], Acta Unio. Intern. Contra Cancrum 19, 80

5. TATARINOV, Yu. S. [1966], Fed. Proc., Transl. Suppl., pt. 2, 25, 344

6. ABELEV, G. I. [1968], Cancer Res. 28, 1344

7. SMITH, J. B. & TODD, D. [1968], Lancet ii, 833

8. ALPERT, M. E., URIEL, J. & DeNECHAUD, B. [1968], N. Engl. J. Med. 278, 984

9. PURVES, L. R., BERSOHN, I. & GEDDES, E. W. [1970], Cancer 25, 1261

10. O'CONOR, G. T., TATARINOV, Yu. S., ABELEV, G. I. & URIEL, J. [1970], Cancer 25, 1091

11. HULL, E. W., CARBONE, P. P., MOERTEL, C. G. & O'CONOR, G. T. [1970], Lancet i, 779

12. SMITH, J. B. & O'NEILL, R. T. [1971], Amer. J. Med. 51, 767

13. SMITH, J. B. [1971], Proc. First Conf. and Workshop on Embryonic and Fetal Antigens in Cancer. Ed. N. G. Anderson and J. Coggin, p. 305

14. ALPERT, E., PINN, V. W. & ISSELBACHER, K. J. [1971], N. Engl. J. Med. 285, 1058

15. KOZOWER, M., FAWAZ, K. A., MILLER, H. M. & KAPLAN, M. M. [1971], N. Engl. J. Med. 285, 1059

16. MEHLMAN, D. J., BULKLEY, B. H. & WIERNIK, P. H. [1971], N. Engl. J. Med. 285, 1060

17. ABELEY,G.I.[1971], In Advances in Cancer Research.Ed. Klein,G. and Weinhouse,S. Academic Press,New York - London, Vol. 14, 295

18. NAYAK,N.C., MALAVIYA,A.N.,CHAWLA,V.& CHANDRA, R.K.[1972], Lancet i, 68

19. SMITH,J.B.[1971], Int.J.Cancer 8, 421

20. RUOSLAHTI,E.& SEPPÄLÄ,M.[1972], Lancet ii,278

21. SMITH,J.B. [1971],Clin.Res. 19,739

22. WALDMANN,T.A. & McINTIRE,K.R.[1972],Lancet ii,1112

23. OLOVNIKOV,A.M. & TSVETKOV,W.S.[1969],Bull.Eksper. Biol.Med. 68, 1426

24. SEPPÄLÄ,M. & RUOSLAHTI,E.[1972],Lancet ii,375

25. PURVES,L.R. & GEDDES,E.W.[1972],Lancet i, 47

26. BROCK,D.J.H. & SUTCLIFFE,R.G.[1972],Lancet ii,197

27. RUOSLAHTI,E.& SEPPÄLÄ,M.[1972],Nature [London] 235,161

28. RUOSLAHTI,E. & SEPPÄLÄ,M.[1971],Int.J.Cancer 8,374

29. NISHI,S.[1970],Cancer Research 30,2507

30. AXEN,R.,PORATH,J. & ERNBACK,S.[1967],Nature [London] 214,1302

31. GREENWOOD,F.C.,HUNTER,W.M. & GLOVER,J.S. [1963],Biochem.J.89, 114

32. ALPERT,E.,STARZL.T.E.,SCHUR,P.H. & ISSELBA- CHER,K.J.[1971],Gastroenterology 61,144

33. AL-SARRAF,M.,KITHIER,K.,POULIK,M.D. & VAITKEVICIUS,V.K. [1971], Clin.Res. 19,647

4.3 Demonstration of Carcinoembryonic Antigens in Tumors of the Gastrointestinal Tract

S. von Kleist

Before starting the subject I shall briefly define what is meant by the term "carcinoembryonic antigens": When in 1965 GOLD and FREEDMAN published their first paper on a cancer specific antigen present in human tumors of the gastrointestinal tract and other organs from the entodermally derived digestive tissue, they coined the expression carcinoembryonic antigen or CEA for this particular substance, because their antigen turned out to be present also in fetal gut, liver, and pancreas up to the 6th month of gestation [1]. Ever since then this denomination has been adopted universally to designate antigens present in malignant and fetal tissues and absent from normal adult organs, as shown principally by the use of hetero-antisera. That this definition is somewhat schematic will be seen later on. At the present time there are 4 carcinoembryonic antigens known in human malignancies, all of which are not rigorously cancer-specific. Two of these antigens are found in primary carcinomas of the digestive tract, i.e. - the CEA of GOLD, which has also been isolated by us, from carcinomas of the colon, the stomach, and their corresponding metastases [2], and

    - the feto-sulphoglycoprotein described by HÄKKINEN to be present in cancerous gastric juice [3].

Another of these antigens is found principally in primary hepatomas, i.e. the α_1FP first described by ABELEV [4] and TATARINOV [5], and the last one has been found quite recently by TROUILLAS in malignant gliomas [6].

One of the two best known antigens is the CEA, which has the
following physico-chemical characteristics:

- it is soluble in 0.6 M perchloric acid,

- it is a glycoprotein with a protein moiety of about 45 %
which is heat resistant,

- it has a sedimentation constant of about 7.2 S and its
molecular weight is generally considered to be 180.000 [7]. It is
easily demonstrable by immunoelectrophoresis or double diffusion reactions in the semipurified, that is acid extracts of intestinal tumors, where it shows up as one of the principal antigens migrating towards the cathode [Fig. 1]. The high sugar
content of the molecule makes it subject to cross reactions with
other glycoproteins, which might interfere with the specific CEA
reaction.

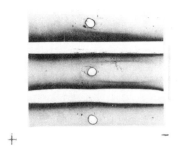

Fig. 1: Immunoelectrophoresis
plate showing in the antigen re-
servoirs [from left to right]:
normal colon extract, purified
CEA, semipurified CEA. In the
antibody troughs [from left to
right]: anti CEA antiserum, anti-
semipurified CEA antiserum. Note
the precipitin line of pure CEA in
the middle and the lines of CEA
and NCA at the right.

By immunofluorescence microscopy the CEA can be demonstrated
abundantly on the luminal surface of the tumor glands specially of
well differenciated epitheliomas of the glandular type [Fig. 2],
whereas in poorly differentiated tumors it becomes less abundant
and anaplastic tumors can be even negative, as has been shown
by DENK et al. [8]. On isolated cells the CEA is distributed all
over the cell surface; GOLD localized it by electronmicroscopy
in the glycocalix of the cell membrane [9]. Gastric tumors as a
whole are less rich in CEA than colonic tumors and microscopic

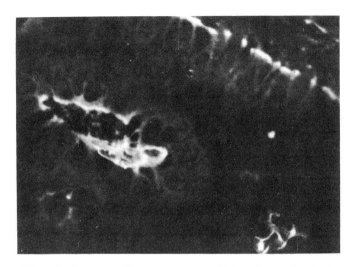

Fig. 2. Immunofluorescence slide of a colonic tumor incubated with anti CEA antiserum . [x 400].

studies done in our laboratory and by DENK and TAPPEINER [8] have confirmed this observation in so far as even well differentiated gastric carcinomas are less frequently highly fluorescent. As has been pointed out by the same authors, the fact, that it needs a well differentiated carcinoma or metastasis in order to get a clear cut result impairs greatly the use of this technique for the identification of undifferentiated metastases of unknown origin. Furthermore, CEA has been shown by us to be present in non cancerous mucosa more than 10 cm off the primary tumor. Similar pictures have been obtained by our group with some well differentiated benign polyps and even with some hemorrhoids [10]. These findings bring about the question of the cancer specificity of the CEA. In normal, that is non inflammatory adult colonic mucosa we have not found appreciable amounts of CEA with the methods we employed. Equal findings have been reported for instance by COLIGAN in TODD's group [11], DENK [8], ØRJASAETER [12] and GOLD [1], of course.

On the other hand there are the absorption experiments of MAR-
TIN and MARTIN which showed the presence of CEA in minute
quantities in normal colonic mucosa extracts, because these
authors could absorb out all specific anti CEA antibodies of any
given immunserum by very large amounts of normal colon extract, thus proving that CEA lacks cancer specificity [13]. Up till
now I have reported results which were exclusively obtained with
heteroimmunsera. The question is, can one demonstrate the CEA
also with autologous sera, in other words, is the CEA autoantigenic? The answer we give to that question is: no! Here we are
in controversy with GOLD, who described only recently again
circulating antibodies directed against CEA in colonic cancer
patients'sera [14]. No one else yet has reproduced his findings.
We have worked for years on this problem but were not able with
any of the various .techniques we tried, i.e. passive hemagglutination, immunoadsorption, immunofluorescence, to demonstrate
anti CEA antibodies. The antibodies we found, - for there are
antibodies, - were all directed against other tumor proteins [15].
Recently LO GERFO has confirmed our negative findings with an
even more sensitive method, the radioimmunoassay [16]. Apparently the CEA does not stimulate cell mediated immunity either,
because when HOLLINGSHEAD and HERBERMAN injected
patients intradermally with soluble fractions of autologous colon
tumor cell membranes they observed positive delayed type hypersensitivity skin reactions. They did not see anything the like
when they injected purified CEA [17]. Likewise, LETENJI in
GOLD's group did not receive any evidence for a cell mediated
immune response either in her test system, which consisted of
patients'lymphocytes blastic transformation upon in vitro exposure to the CEA [18]. Of course one might argue that the CEA in
vivo contains a protein constituent which permits the stimulation

of both cell mediated and humoral immunity and that the acid
extraction removes part of the protein or alters the sugars, thus
leaving behind a molecule, which no longer stimulates cell mediated immunity. This brings about still another problem: that of
the possible differences between the native and the extracted
antigen, and as far as the native is concerned, the still fixed and
the circulating antigen, which is traced by the radioimmunoassay.
For the CEA circulates in the serum of tumor bearing patients,
but only in nanogram quantities, so that it needs the highly sensitive radioimmunoassay in order to trace it. Unfortunately also
only advanced cancers release sufficient CEA to be traced even
by this method. I shall not go into this any further as this will
be treated elsewhere.

I shall now turn briefly to the two other colon tumor antigens
which I mentioned at the beginning because in a way they are also
carcinofetal antigens because present both in fetal and tumor
tissues. The one with ß electrophoretic mobility is the antigen
we recently isolated also from hepatic metastases of colonic
carcinomas [19]. It is also a perchlorosoluble glycoprotein, but
of considerably smaller molecular size [3 - 4 S], which permits
its separation from CEA preparations of which it is a tenacious
contaminant by gel filtration. The most striking feature is the
fact, that it crossreacts immunologically with anti CEA antibodies thus giving a reaction of partial identity in the double diffusion test [Fig. 3].

We found the antigen present in appreciable amounts in normal
tissues [lung, spleen]. It is hence neither organ nor cancer specific and we named it therefore non specific crossreacting antigen
or NCA. There are, besides the common part, different specific
antigenic determinants on each molecule: in the case of NCA

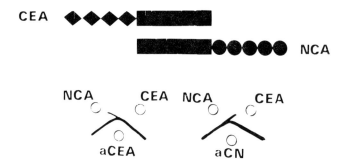

Fig. 3. Schema illustrating the partial identity of the CEA and NCA molecules and the double diffusion reactions demonstrating the same phenomenon. aCN = anti normal colonic mucosa antiserum.

tested with an aCEA and pure CEA the spur indicates specific unshared sites on the CEA molecule, while when an antiserum against normal colon mucosa extract was employed the spur indicates this time the presence of a specific antigenic site on the NCA molecule. This proves that the NCA is not simply a fragment of the CEA molecule. Eventual practical implications of this for the CEA tests are treated elsewhere.

The α antigen is also a fetal protein, which is, as has been shown by COLLATZ in our laboratory, autoantigenic. It is for this reason that it deserves special interest. Part of the circulating antibodies found in tumor patients' sera are directed against this particular component. It is also a cell membrane associated antigen as is the CEA and NCA. The NCA has a similar fluorescent pattern than the CEA, except for marked staining of all the cell contoures which is characteristic for NCA. The α antigen apparently is localized both in the cytoplasm and the membrane.

I shall finish now by mentioning the second carcinoembryonic antigen of the digestive tract, the feto-sulphoglycoprotein or FSA of HÄKKINEN. This substance is demonstrated by immunofluorescence in fetal stomach mucosa and gastric carcinomas with heteroimmunsera prepared against a sulphoglycoprotein isolated from gastric juice of gastric cancer patients. The cancer specificity of this substance is somewhat obscured by the fact that by the OUCHTERLONY technique the antigen can be demonstrated also in the juice of a few cases of peptic ulcer juice and in aged patients'normal gastric juice. Recently HÄKKINEN has published a paper [20] indicating that his antigen is part of the CEA, in other words there is still another substance which reacts with anti CEA antibodies. HÄKKINEN's work has not yet been reproduced in other laboratories, but we are currently investigating on the identity of NCA and FSA.

References

1. GOLD,P. & FREEDMAN,S.[1965],J.Exp.Med.121,439

2. von KLEIST,S. & BURTIN,P.[1969],Cancer Res. 29,1961

3. HÄKKINEN,I.,JARVI,O. & GROUROOS,J.[1968],Int.J. Cancer, 3, 572

4. ABELEV,G.,PEROVA,S.,KRAMKOVA,N.,POSTNIKOVA,Z. & IRLIN,I. [1963], Transplantation 1, 174

5. TATARINOV,Yu. [1964],I.Biochem.Congress [USSR] [Abstracts] 2, 274

6. TROUILLAS,P. [1971], Lancet 2, 552

7. KRUPEY,J.,GOLD,Ph. & FREEDMAN,S.[1968],J.Exp. Med. 128, 387

8. DENK,H.,TAPPEINER,G.,ECKESTORFER,R. & HOLZNER,J.H.[1972],Int.J.Cancer 10,262

9. GOLD,P.,GOLD,M. & FREEDMAN,S.[1968],Cancer Res. 28,1331

10. BURTIN, P., MARTIN, E., SABINE, M.C. & von KLEIST, S. [1972], J.Nat.Cancer Inst. 48, 25

11. COLIGAN, J.E., LAUTENSCHLEGER, J.T., EGAN, M.L. & TODD, C.W.[1972], Immunochemistry 9, 377

12. ØRJASAETER, H., FREDRIKSEN, G. and LIAVAG, I.[1972], Acta Path.Microbiol.Scand.Section B 80, 599

13. MARTIN, F. & MARTIN, M.S. [1970], Int.J.Cancer 6, 352

14. GOLD, J.M., FREEDMAN, S. & GOLD, P.[1972], Nature New Biol. 239, 60

15. COLLATZ, E., von KLEIST, S. & BURTIN, P.[1971], Int.J. Cancer 8, 298

16. LO GERFO, P., HERBER, F.P. & BENNETT, S.J.[1972], Int.J.Cancer 9, 344

17. HOLLINSHEAD, A., MacWRIGHT, C., ALFORD, T., GLEW, D., GOLD, P. & HERBERMAN, R.[1972], Science 177, 887

18. LEJTENJI, M.C., FREEDMAN, S. & GOLD, P.[1971], Cancer 28, 115

19. von KLEIST, S., CHAVANEL, G. & BURTIN, P. [1972], P.N.A.S. [U.S.A.], 69, 2492

20. HÄKKINEN, I. [1972], Immunochemistry 9, 115

4.4 Radioimmunoassay of CEA: Its Use in Diagnosis and Prognosis of Human Carcinoma

G. Pusztaszeri and J.-P. Mach

The problem of the specificity of the radioimmunoassay of CEA for the diagnosis of carcinoma of the digestive tract has been lately the subject of a great controversy [1, 2, 3]. The purpose of our work was to establish if it was possible to find back the specificity of the radioimmunoassay of CEA for digestive carcinoma originally described by GOLD. Special care was taken to absorb the anti-CEA antiserum with large amounts of the normal glycoprotein crossreacting with CEA [4].

We employed the same technique as GOLD [1], using his goat G-81 anti-CEA antiserum absorbed with perchloric acid extracts of normal lung, liver and gut, at a ratio of 50 mg/ml of each.

Out of 100 cases of digestive carcinoma, 68 had a plasma CEA value over the arbitrary limit of 5 ng/ml. Sixty seven percent of the cases of bronchial carcinoma and 45% of those of mammary carcinoma showed CEA levels above this limit. Furthermore, 43 % of the patients with non cancerous digestive diseases had a plasma CEA level over 5 ng/ml; most of these patients had ulcerative colitis. If the cases of digestive carcinoma are separated into 2 groups, according to the estimated size of the tumor and its degree of spreading, it appears that only 49% of those with tumors smaller than 100 cc, and only locally invasive had a plasma CEA level above 5 ng/ml, whereas 87% of those with larger tumors, or with distant metastases were above this level. A significant difference was observed in post-operative CEA levels between the patients having undergone a complete resection of their tumor and those in which only partial resection was possible. Out of the 19 cases of the first category, 14 had normal levels before surgery, which remained unchanged, the 5 other cases who had elevated levels before surgery all showed a drop to normal CEA levels within 2 to 3 weeks after complete resection. In patients of the second category, the plasma CEA levels remained elevated after surgery.

In spite of a thorough absorption of the anti-CEA antiserum with the normal glycoprotein crossreacting with CEA, we did not obtain a test specific for digestive carcinoma [5]. An explanation of the non specificity of the radioimmunoassay of CEA was given since we were able to identify CEA in tissue extracts from bronchial carcinoma, mammary carcinoma, and in much smaller amounts in normal lung [6]. The presence of CEA appears thus not to be restricted only to the entodermally derived organs, as previously thought.

At the present time, the usefullness of the CEA test for the early diagnosis of carcinoma seems to be quite limited, but it can be considered as suggesting the presence of a carcinoma when the CEA level is elevated above 10 to 20 ng/ml, in the absence of any alternative pathological condition. One of the most promising applications of the CEA test appears to be in the follow-up of patients with a known carcinoma.

References

1. THOMPSON, D. M. P. , KRUPEY, J. , FREEDMAN, S. O. & GOLD, P. [1969], Proc. Nat. Acad. Sci. USA 64, 161

2. LO GERFO, P. , KRUPEY, J. & HANSEN, H. J. [1971], N. Engl. J. Med. 285, 138

3. ZAMCHECK, N. , MOORE, T. L. , DHAR, P. & KUPCHIK, H. Z. [1972], N. Engl. J. Med. 286, 83

4.   MACH, J.-P. & PUSZTASZERI, G. [1972], Immunochemistry 9, 1031

5.   MACH, J.-P., PUSZTASZERI, G., DYSLI, M., KAPP, F.,
     BIERENS DE HAAN, B., LOOSLI, R.M., GROB, P. &
     ISLIKER, H. [1973], Schweiz. Med. Wochenschr. [in press]

6.   PUSZTASZERI, G. & MACH, J.-P. [1974], Immunochemistry [in press]

4.5 A Contribution for the Detection of Fetal Antigens in Serum of Tumor Patients[1]

H. Schultze-Mosgau and K. Fischer

The detection of fetal antigens is becoming increasingly important in the diagnosis of tumors (1-7).

Since it is known that certain tumors carry antigens which are
normally restricted to the fetal period, we immunized rabbits
with placenta antigens, and obtained 3 different precipitins
which did not react with a normal adult serum. An extract was
prepared (8) from placentae from normal pregnancies where both
mother and child had blood group 0. The placentae were rinsed
with prewarmed (37°C) isotonic NaCl solutions to remove most
of the blood. After the perfusion, an equal volume of isotonic
NaCl solution was added to the placentae, which were then minced
in a Starmix. The mixture was homogenized in an Ultra-Turrax
mixer and separated by centrifugation (10 min at 1800 x g) into
sedimented placenta stroma and soluble placenta extract. The
macromolecular and aggregated placenta proteins were obtained
by further centrifugation of the soluble placenta extract in an
ultracentrifuge (1 h at 100 000 x g). The sediment obtained in this
way was redissolved in isotonic NaCl solution and brought to a
protein concentration of 1g/100 ml (Biuret determination).

The anti-placenta serum (8) was produced by injecting rabbits
parenterally at three- to four-week intervals with 0. 5 ml of the
1 perc. placenta protein solution, in some cases mixed with
FREUND's adjuvant complete. The rabbit sera were tested for

1) Supported by a grant from the Deutsche Forschungsgemeinschaft.

precipitating antibodies with the OUCHTERLONY technique (9) and immunoelectrophoresis (10). At the end of the immunization period, the antisera were mixed in a ratio of 5 to 6 with human serum from healthy donors of various blood groups in order to eliminate antibodies against human plasma proteins. To prevent cross reactions, the rabbit antisera were also incubated with an excess of dried kidney and liver tissue.

Figure 1 shows the precipitation lines with placenta extract. A weakly precipitating fraction moves most rapidly toward the anode. The most slowly moving fraction is somewhat more heavily precipitated. The third, particularly heavy precipitation line is found in the middle. Although the anti-placenta serum reacted negatively in the OUCHTERLONY test with the sera of 50 healthy blood donors, we found two precipitation lines in the serum of each of 30 women at the end of pregnancy (Fig. 2).

+   –

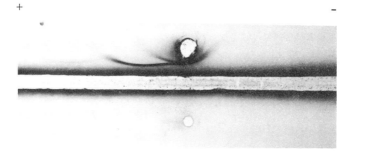

Placenta

Anti-pla-
centa serum

Normal
serum

Fig. 1. Reaction of absorbed rabbit anti-placenta serum with electrophoretically separated placenta extract or blood-donor serum.
Separation time 60 min, constant voltage 5 V/cm, barbiturate buffer pH 8.6, ionic strength 0.037, immunodiffusion time 48 h.

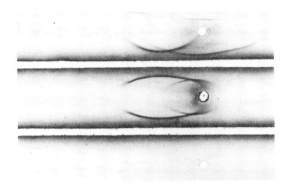

Serum of pregnant woman

Anti-placenta serum

Placenta

Anti-placenta serum

Normal serum

Fig. 2. Reaction of absorbed anti-placenta serum with electrophoretically separated serum of pregnant woman and
placenta extract.
Experimental conditions as in Figure 1.

Positive reactions with anti-placenta serum were also observed
with the blood of newborns, the amniotic fluid and the ascites of
hydropic newborns. The appropriate electrophoretic comparisons
showed that specific proteohormones like FSH, HCG human fibrinogen and hemoglobin were not involved. The anti-placenta
serum did not precipitate the α_1-feto-protein or the C-reactive
protein. However, a weak precipitation line appears if the anti-
placenta serum is allowed to react with an extract of Fallopian
tubes or endometrium. In the serum of these women, however,
there were no fetal antigens which could be detected by the
OUCHTERLONY test. Ovarian and myometrium extracts did not
react. The fetal antigens which react with the anti-placenta
serum were sometimes found in the sera of women with cancerous and benign tumors. The precipitation lines from the reaction
of anti-placenta serum with the serum of a patient with a metastasizing ovarian carcinoma are shown in Figure 3. A corresponding reaction is seen with the tumor itself, but there is no
reaction with normal ovarian tissue or normal donor serum.

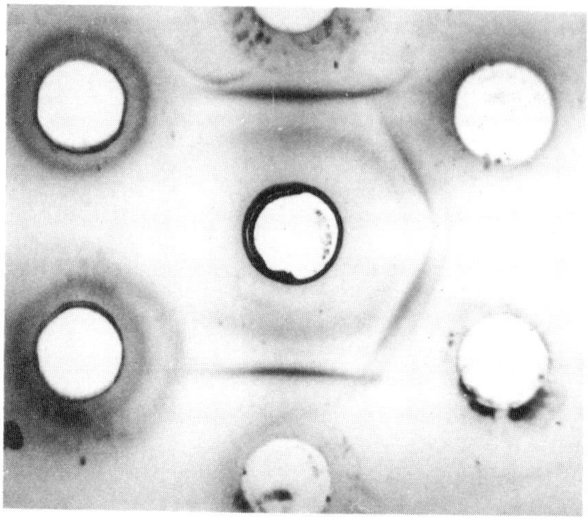

Placenta

Fig. 3. Reaction of anti-placenta serum with the sera of patients with ovarial carcinoma and ovarial tumor, normal ovarial tissue and normal donor serum. Immunodiffusion time 48 h.

The three precipitated tumor proteins were shown by immuno-electrophoresis to be identical to the three placenta antigens. The placenta antigens discussed here are found not only in the case of malignant ovarian tumors, but also in the sera of patients with cervical carcinoma, corpus carcinoma, mammary carcinoma, malignant dysgerminoma and chorionic epithelioma. We found no placenta antigens in the sera of children with leukemia (3 acute, 2 chronic). The following table (Tab. 1) summarizes the cases which have been examined to date with the OUCHTERLONY technique.

The high percentage of positive reactions in cases of ovarial carcinomas is striking. There was no recognizable correlation between the presence of individual precipitation lines and the

Table 1:

Positive reactions of treated rabbit anti-placenta
serum with sera from tumor patients

Tumor	No.	Positive reaction
Mammary carcinoma	53	11 (21%)
Cervical carcinoma	40	5 (13%)
Vulva, vaginal carc.	18	5 (27%)
Ovarian carcinoma	16	7 (44%)
Corpus carcinoma	12	3 (25%)
Malign. dysgerminoma	1	1
Chorionic epithelioma	1	1
Hydatide mole	2	2
Leukemia	5	-
Pregnant women	30	30 (100%)
Normal	50	- (0 %)

type of tumor, so it cannot be decided whether the tumor cells
synthesize the fetal proteins and excrete them into the plasma.
It is possible that the tumors produce substances which stimulate
the organism to synthesize the fetal proteins. That this ability
is not lost after the fetal period can be seen from the fact that
in various hematological disorders, for example thalassemia,
erythrocytes containing hemoglobin-F are found, often in large
numbers. Another indication is the failure of adults to form antibodies against fetal antigens from the same species. This suggests a tolerance which is maintained by the continued presence
of small amounts of fetal antigens (maintenance of tolerance).

We would call for the establishment of reference laboratories which would make possible the classification of the fetal antigens found in many different places.

References

1. ALEXANDER, P. (1972), Nature(London) 235, 137

2. PEDERSEN, K. O. (1944), Nature (London) 144, 575

3. OETTGEN, H. F. (1970), 2. Tagg. Ges. Immunol., Wien

4. O'CONOR, G. T. & URIEL, J. (1971), Cancer Res. 25, 1091

5. GOLD, P., GOLD, M. & FREEDMAN, S. O. (1968), Cancer Res. 28, 1331

6. ABELEV, G. (1970), 18th Coll. Protides Biol. Fluids, Brügge

7. EDYNAK, E. M., OLD, L. J., VRANA, M. & LARDIS, M. (1970), Proc. Amer. Assoc. Cancer Res. 11, 22

8. SCHULTZE-MOSGAU, H. & FISCHER, K. (1971), Arch. Gynäkol. 210, 458

9. OUCHTERLONY, Ö. (1949), Acta Pathol. Microbiol. Scand. 26, 516

10. GRABAR, P. & WILLIAMS, C. A. (1953), Biochim. Biophys. Acta (Amsterdam) 10, 193

5 Methods for Detection of Proteins Excreted by Tumor Cells

5.1 Experiments to Induce Myeloma Protein-Forming Neoplasma in Rodents

G. Hermann

In the experimental induction of plasma-cellular tumors in mice 3 important problems are combined:

1. The effect of oil in water emulsions, which simultaneously potentiate the immune response, upon the lympho-reticular system.

2. The transformation into tumoral cells of a cell capable of producing antibodies.

3. The generation of myeloma proteins or BENCE-JONES proteins in isohistogeneous animal strains.

In addition the possible viral origin of the plasmocytomas or plasmosarcomas and probably genetic factors must be considered.

FREUND's type adjuvant (1,2,3) exactly like its individual components, has, besides its known stimulatory effect upon the immune response, a particular affinity to the lympho-reticular system. Intensity of the reaction and effect depends on the method of application and the species of animal. In mice, the small lymphocytes disappear and the reticulum cells proliferate after the introduction of adjuvants into lymphnodes and the spleen 4 . The secondary changes show gradual differences which were strongest with complete adjuvants, less strong with incomplete adjuvants and least strong after the injection of the mineral oil component (5). After intraperitoneal injection a proliferous activity among the reticulo- endothelial cells with mononuclear and histiocytic infiltration of the portal areas in the liver was found, and in the spleen a proliferation of the red pulp with plasma cells, histiocytes

and numerous giant cells was visible. After intravenous injection
(7) the changes occur predominantly in the spleen, because the
spleen acts as a filter for the blood circulation. After subcutaneous injections of complete FREUND's type adjuvants, hypochro-
matic macrocytic anaemias with reticulocytosis, leucocytosis with
relative lymphopenia and hyperplasias with an increased number
of erythroblasts in the bone marrow were apparent.

These experiments indicate that after the injection of adjuvants
or mineral oil, "irritations" of the lymphoreticular system occur
which, on the one hand, lead to a prolongation of the immune response, and on the other, favour the formation of tumors of this
cell system.

Plasma-cell leukaemias and a plasma-cellular tumor were described by RASK-NIELSEN and GORMSEN (9) in mice of the
strain STREET, by BICHEL (10) in a mouse of the strain AK, by
DUNN (11) in mice of the strain C3H and by MERVIN and ALGIRE
(12) for the first time in the mouse strain BALB/c. Plasma-cell
leukaemias and plasmocytomas had appeared, partly after the
injection of cancerogeneous substances benzpyrene, di-benzan-
thracene or methylcholanthrene (9), either spontaneously or following the implantation of diffusion chambers with mamma-tumors.
A viral factor was suspected, as spontaneous plasma-cell tumors
in BALB/c mice had not been observed, but nevertheless some
tumors did appear even after the intraperitoneal implantation of
empty diffusion chambers.

Furthermore POTTER and KUFF (13) described the development
of plasma-cell tumors in BALB/c mice after the intraperitoneal
injection of paraffin oil, adjuvants and heat-killed staphylococci
mixtures. In this way a possibility seemed open for the extensive
induction of plasma-cellular-tumors.

The following is a description of our experiments to induce plasma-cellular tumors with Bayol F in various strains of mice and in rats of the strain WISTAR/HAN.

Material and Methods

193 mice of the strain BALB/c, 62 mice of the strain IC (Institut du Cancer), 42 mice of the strain C3H, 10 mice of the strain S42 and 10 DBA-2 were arranged in several series and received injections of Bayol F in varying quantities and at various intervals of time. The animals were kept under observation for a minimum of 24 months.

147 rats of the strain WISTAR/HAN, maintained under SPF (specific pathogen free) conditions, received at various times 3 injections of Bayol F, in every case at intervals of one week. 24 animals were kept under observation for 38 weeks, 12 for 21 months.

The clear, transparent paraffin oil injected is a mineral oil with the designation Bayol 55 (or Bayol F) and was obtained from the Esso International Corporation, New York 20, N.Y. The oil contains no aromatic substances.

Simple agarelectrophoreses and immunoelectrophoreses were carried out after the fashion of GRABAR and WILLIAMS (14-16) partly in the micromodification according to SCHEIDEGGER (17).

The following immune sera from rabbits were used:
Polyspecific antisera: anti-mouse serumproteins and anti-mouse urineproteins. Bispecific sera: anti-mouse transferrin and anti-mouse immunoglobulin G; anti-mouse immunoglobulin G and anti-mouse immunoglobulin M.

<u>Monospecific antisera</u>: anti-mouse immunoglobulin A and fluoresceine isocyanate-marked monospecific anti-mouse IgA.

For the electron microscope photographs of plasmocytomas I have to thank Madame Nicole GRANBOULAN, Institut de Recherches Scientifiques sur le Cancer, Villejuif (Val de Marne), France.

Results

1. As regards the electrophoretic mobility of single fractions, there exist no differences between human serum and mouse serum, only the gamma globulin fraction in the mouse migrates comparatively faster. But considerable differences arise in the percentage sub-division of the individual fractions. In comparison with human serum, mouse serum contains less albumin (43, 9%) more α_1 globulins (17, 5%), less α_2 globulins (4, 3%), less β_1 globulins (4, 8%), significantly more β_2 globulins (18, 7%) and very few gamma globulins (3, 5%) (Fig. 1 and 2).

In the immunoelectrophoretic analysis a good anti-mouse serum reveals 16-18 lines of precipitation.

Apart from the immunoglobulins, approximately 12 serum globulins in mice have been more closely identified. CLAUSEN and HEREMANS (18) have drawn up a serviceable working nomenclature which we were able to retain in part. As yet there exists no binding international nomenclature for the designation of the serum of laboratory animals because, astonishingly, some fundamental data necessary for its determination are still unknown (19). There is however widespread agreement on the immunoglobulins of mice, despite their varying nomenclature. Those commonly accepted are IgG_2, IgG_1, IgM and IgA as well as subgroups of the immunoglobulin class IgG.

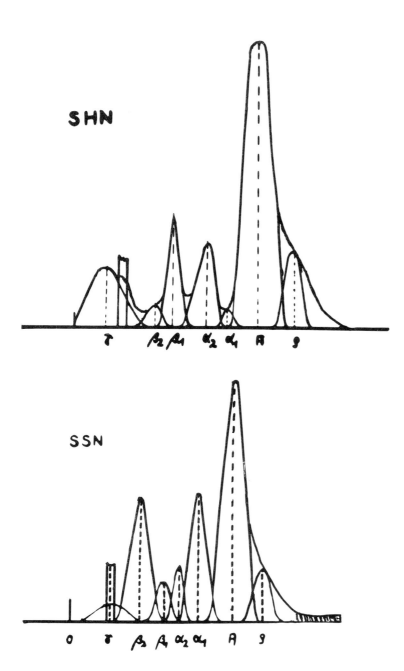

Fig. 1 and 2. Extinction curves of bromphenolblue-stained agar-
electrophoresis of fresh normal human (NHS) and
normal mouse serum (NMS).

The serum proteins of rats are less well known, probably because there have been scarcely any myeloma noted in this species. However, the immunoglobulins IgG_2, IgG_1, IgA and IgM have been identified and the preparations and effects of monospecific antisera recorded (20). Anti-mouse IgG_2 shows cross-reactions with rat IgG (21). Since anti-IgA serum for mice cross-reacts with rat IgA, all 4 immunoglobulins of rats can be specified and determined.

The Paraffinoma

We were able to distinguish 3 stages in the generation of the paraffinoma in mice:

1. After the injection of Bayol F the quantity of mononuclear cells and macrophages normally present in small numbers in the peritoneal cavity of the mouse increases sharply in a matter of a few days. Plasmocytes also appear (Stage 1). Subsequently pale white nodules form in the immediate vicinity of the small blood vessels and of the lymph canals. They contain Bayol F, grow larger in the course of repeated injections and are localized over the whole visceral peritoneum. The vascularization of the mesenterium increases. The intestines have scarcely ever been conspicuously affected, the paraffinoma nodules appear in great number on the mesosthenium and in the ligaments. The speed and nature of the development of the nodules and the fibrous tissue depend on the quantity and frequency of the paraffin oil injections.

The nodules contain mononuclear basophilic cells, fibroblasts, macrophages and plasma cells. The accumulation of oil causes the macrophages to assume bizarre shapes. As a result of the reaction to foreign bodies multiple-nuclear cells, mononuclear cells with karyorrhexis and karyolysis are occasionally found.

This persistent destruction of cells and the constant phagocytosis of cell remains and non-metabolizable paraffin oil maintains a consistent state of irritation. In mice at 16, 20 and 24 weeks after the first injection, fragmentations and double, triple and occasionally quadruple expansions of IgG_2 precipitation lines in the immuno-electrophoresis develop. Sub-groups of the immunoglobulin γ_2 now seem to appear quite plainly. But in 2 out of 3 of the animals examined a temporary hypo-γ globulinaemia can be detected. The immune response of the precipitating antibodies after the injection of ovalbumin is, however, increased (22). In mice of the strain BALB/c paraffin oil injections in subcutaneously-made air-pockets lead neither to paraffinomas nor to tumors.

The paraffinoma develops in rats in the same way as in mice. Macrophages, histiocytes and plasma cells are present in microscopic examination, storing the mineral oil in the cytoplasma and occasionally in small vacuoles in the cell nucleus (Fig. 3). The paraffin granuloma is most strongly visible after 12 weeks. After 21 months however, still only minute paraffinoma nodules were to be found on the visceral peritoneum of the liver and the spleen, while the whole mesenterium was unaffected.

In contrast with mice, rats can apparently metabolize, break down or excrete paraffin oil. Rats do not display hypo-γ globulinemia, but a clearly augmented immune response of the haemolysin forming cells after the injection of sheep erythrocytes, as long as the paraffinoma remains (23).

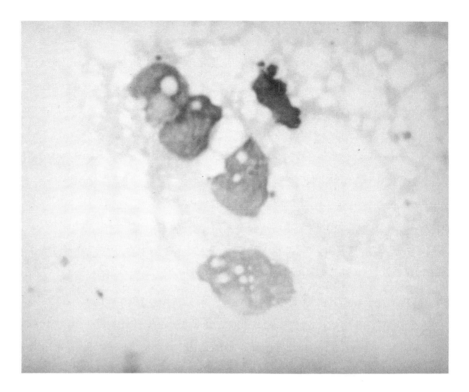

Fig. 3. Crush preparation of an paraffinoma nodule from WISTAR/
HAN rat. Panoptic staining PAPPENHEIM.
Magnification 2000 : 1. 2 histiocytes and 2 plasmocyte-
like cells with large vacuols in nuclei and protoplasma.

Frequency of the Tumors

Out of 193 mice of the strain BALB/c injected with Bayol F 42
(21, 8%) developed a pathological condition. In 31 cases (16, 1%)
an ascites with erythrocytes and abnormal plasmocytes appeared,
in 11 cases (5, 7%) not only a plasmocytic haemorrhagic ascites,
but also localized tumors occured. There was one non-haemor-
rhagic ascites and in one case a liver-adenoma was found. 48
animals under supervision showed no pathological signs over an
observation period of 20 or more months. The sharply fluctuat-
ing figures in the various series of the experiments do not permit

any conclusions to be drawn as to the effectiveness of one or the
other of the injection methods. But, like POTTER (24), we did
obtain the highest number of tumors with 4 injections of 0, 5 ml
Bayol F at bi-monthly intervals.

The earliest occurence of haemorrhagic plasmocytic ascites was
observed in two cases 5 months after the first injection of Bayol F.
The first tumor appeared in the 7th month. Tumors and pathological ascites appear most frequently in the 11th month. The majority
of pathological symptoms come to light from the 9th to the 13th
month. From the 18th month onwards only the sporadic appearance
of further tumors can be expected (25) (Fig. 4).

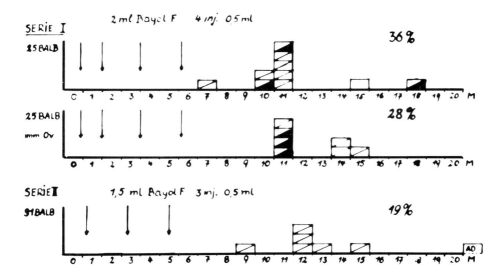

Fig. 4. Frequency of the tumors and plasmocytic haemorrhagic
ascites in 3 series of mice injected with Bayol F.

In the rats no transformation into plasma-cellular tumors took place, possibly because the paraffinoma does not persist.

Morphology of the Tumors

a. Ascites

The externally visible form of an ascites after the lapse of 5-9 weeks shows the nature of tumor growth. An autopsy reveals up to 20-25 ml haemorrhagic ascites. Only 1 out of 3 animals exhibits a localized tumor the size of a pin-head to that of a pea. The dark red tumors are almost always localized on the mesenterium. The ascites contains numerous plasmocytes or plasmoblasts and only very few lymphatic elements. The quantity of leucocytes per mm^3 exceeds the amount of white corpuscles in the blood by 2 to 3 times. If the ascites develops late, in other words 12 or more months after the first injection of Bayol F, there are relatively more lymphocytes to be found than in the case of early developed ascites forms, and the sum total of white cells is only slightly more than that of the leucocytes in the blood. In addition to macrophages, which often contain 2 - 3 nucleoli, there are numerous epithelial cells and few granulocytes present.

Binuclear plasmocytes are abundant. The tumorous plasma cells display sharply differing stages of development. There are frequent instances of cells with probably oil containing vacuoles in their nuclei and in isolated fragments split nuclei can be found. This karyorrhexis may be partly attributed to the fact that the cells exhaust and destroy themselves in the attempt to metabolize the paraffin oil, or it may be a sign of malignancy.

b. Solid Tumors

The solid tumors occur in the granulation tissue (Fig. 5). The fibrous capsules of the organ are thicker, and plasmocytomas appeared in nodules on the liver and kidney capsules. Even in impression preparations of paraffin oil nodules incipient accumulations were found which already showed a tendency towards tumor development.

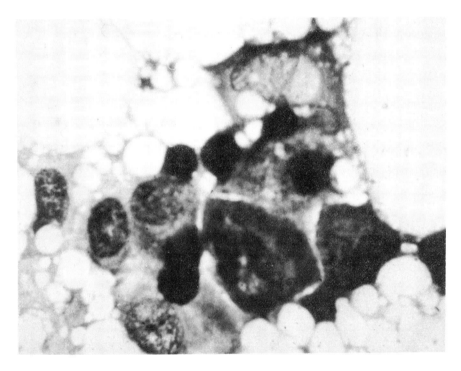

Fig. 5. Early state of a plasma cell cluster in the granulation tissue, most probably tumor cells. Panoptic staining according to PAPPENHEIM.

Histologically it is a question in almost all cases of typical plasmosarcomas. From case to case the cells differ to a greater or lesser extent, as proplasmoblasts, plasmoblasts and in part almost complete plasmocytes are found. Only in a small proportion of the primary tumors could pathological plasma cells be found in the spleen. The bone marrow was normal in all the cases examined.

In contrast to KAHLER's type disease in humans, there exists primarily no affinity to the bone marrow in the plasmosarcomas of the mouse.

After the injection of plasmatumoral ascites cells into the peritoneal cavity of isohistogeneous BALB/c mice, only solid tumors occur. Solid tumors and tumoral ascites cells could equally be transplanted subcutaneously, in which case local tumors would arise. The predominant result of the intravenous injection of tumoral plasmocytes is bone lesions which resemble KAHLER's type disease in humans. There does exist here, therefore, a definitive affinity to the bone marrow.

The disease that can be generated in experimental animals corresponds therefore almost completely with its human equivalent.

One may therefore also draw the conclusion that "multiple myeloma" results, from one transformed tumor cell, and that the almost always supervised occurrences in humans are metastases. This is unequivocally supported by the fact that myeloma proteins, or BENCE-JONES proteins, are monoclonal. We only know of one observation by POTTER where he found 2 primary tumors in the same animal producing myeloma globulin belonging to two different classes of immunoglobulins.The primary tumors could be trans - planted separately into recipient mice of the same strain; and 2 different tumor lines developed, producing different myeloma proteins.

Myeloma and BENCE-JONES Proteins in Induced Plasmocytomas

Myeloma or BENCE-JONES proteins could be detected easily in the ascites, somewhat less easily in the serum. Barely any differences in the immunoelectrophoresis of ascites and serum can be detected, and then not until the pathological condition is fully developed.

Myeloma globulin belonging to the class G of immunoglobulin occured most frequently, among which, typically, slow-moving, medium-fast-moving and fast-moving myeloma globulin with partial identity to IgG were observed (Fig. 6).

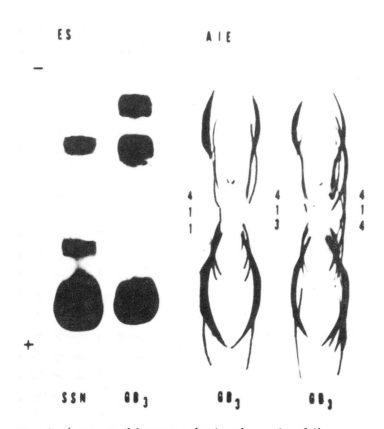

Fig. 6. Agar- and immunoelectrophoresis of the serum of a γ -plasmocytoma-bearing mouse. The different antisera reveal different patterns.

Myeloma globulin of the type IgM or IgA were seldom seen, and constituted roughly 4 - 8 % of the frequency of changes from IgG. Rarer still are multiple changes. The serum of the mouse IJ 5 revealed under immunoelectrophoresis a myeloma protein of the type IgG and a double-curved quantitatively augmented IgM line of precipitation. The question whether there were two primary tumors present forming different myeloma globulins could not be determined. Occasionally, but by no means in all cases, BENCE-JONES proteins are found excreted in the urine. They are detectable through antisera prepared for use against mouse serum proteins, and partly also through antisera for use against mouse urinary proteins. FANTINI, CATTANEO and INVERNIZZI (26) were able to identify a kryoglobulinaemia of the type IgM in a plasmocytoma which had likewise been induced through the intraperitoneal injection of Bayol F in a BALB/c mouse.

Only approximately 10 % of the tumors induced successfully take in animals of the same strain after transplantation and effect the beginning of transplantation lines.

It seems worth noting that after the first transplantation the solitary tumors only develop after a lapse of several weeks or months, and in 4-5 further transplants the ratio of successful takes and the time of development become shorter, until constant ratios result. The ratio of successful takes is then 100%; the length of time from the inoculation of the tumor to the death of the animal in the experiment is very constant. Whether questions of iso-immunity are relevant here is something we have not investigated, but we consider it a possibility. The characteristics of the tumor and the myeloma proteins remain unchanged. Several tumors were transplanted 80 - 100 times; occasionally a sudden unaccountable loss of myeloma protein formation occured.

We observed a leuco-lympho-sarcoma which was the starting-point of one transplantation line. Apart from that, 2 sarcomas appeared, in one of which a characteristic decrease in the immunoglobulin IgA took place.

Mice of the strain IC, the strain C3H, the strain S42 and the strain DBA2 developed a distinct paraffinoma. Only one mouse of the strain DBA2 developed a fibrosarcoma, which we regard as having grown spontaneously. One mouse of the strain C3H developed a plasmosarcoma and exhibited a paraprotein of the type immunoglobulin A (Previously labeled IgY).

All the rats examined developed a paraffinoma but no plasmocytoma, which we connect with the later retrogression of the paraffinoma. Since the time the colloquium was held BAZIN, DECKERS, BECKERS and HEREMANS (27 - 38) described a transplantable immunoglobulin-secreting tumor in rats of the strain LOU/Wsl. A shortened list of the interesting discovery and the results published by these authors is given to the references.

Electron Microscope Examinations

All the plasma cells taken from ascites fluid or the tumor cells taken from solid tumors examined revealed virus-like particles adhering to the endoplasmatic reticulum of the plasma cells.

Summary

On the strength of long-standing examinations, we come to the conclusion that the injection of paraffin oil does offer a possibility of producing experimental plasmosarcomas. The plasmocytic tumors form myeloma proteins which can be assigned to all known immunoglobulin classes. Furthermore, a leuco-lympho-sarcoma and two polymorphous sarcomas were observed. But the possi-

bility of induction is largely confined to mice of the strain BALB/c.
A tumor growth in a mouse of the strain DBA2, as well as earlier
recorded spontaneous or induced tumors, indicates that such tumors could perhaps also be produced in other mouse strains,
given large enough experimental programs. In contrast to mice,
the paraffinoma in rats shows retrogression after several months.
Plasmocytomas were not found. This goal, particularly important
because a further clarification of rat immunoglobulin might have
ensued, can possibly be achieved by another means of injection.
Bayol F seems not to be a cancerogeneous substance in the strict
sense of the word. The examinations indicate that not only viral
but also genetic factors may affect the histological type and the
generation of the plasmosarcomas in mice.

1. The experiments were partly carried out in collaboration with
G. LESPINATS and R. DERNBACH.
2. Partly subsidized by the Government Department for Research,
Nordrhein-Westfalen. Grant Nr. 5203.

References

1. FREUND, J. & BONATO, M. V. (1944), J. Immunol. 48, 325

2. FREUND, J. & McDERMOTT, K. (1942), Proc. Soc. Exp. Biol.
    Med. 49, 548

3. FREUND, J. , THOMSON, K. , HOUGH, H. B. , SOMMER, H. E. &
    PISANI, T. M. (1948), J. Immunol. 60, 383

4. SCHENK, K. E. & MANSKOPF, G. (1968), Beitr. Pathol. Anat.
    137, 391

5. LAUFER, A. , ROSEMANN, E. & DAVIES, A. M. (1966), Brit.
    J. Exp. Pathol. 47, 605

6. LAUFER, A. , TAL, C. & BEHAR, A. J. (1959), Brit. J. Exp.
    Pathol. 40, 1

7. GONET, A. , RUTISHAUSER, E. , WIDGREN, A. & ENGELHORN, A. (1960), Med. Exp. 3, 336

8. MIKOLAJEW, M. , KURATOWSKA, Z. , KOSSAKOWSKA, M. , PLACHECKA, M. & KOPEC, M. (1969), Ann. Rheum. Dis. 28, 35

9. RASK-NIELSEN, R. & GORMSEN, H. (1951), Cancer 4, 387

10. BICHEL, J. (1951), Acta Pathol. Microbiol. Scand. 29, 464

11. DUNN, T. B. (1954), Proc. Amer. Ass. Cancer Res. 1, 13

12. MERVIN, R. M. & ALGIRE, G. H. (1959), Proc. Soc. Exp. Biol. USA 101, 437

13. POTTER, M. & KUFF, E. L. (1961), J. Nat. Cancer Inst. 26, 1109

14. GRABAR, P. & WILLIAMS, C. A. jr. (1953), Biochim. Biophys. Acta 17, 67

15. GRABAR, P. & BURTIN, P. (1964), Immunelektrophoretische Analyse, p. 134, Elsevier Publishing Company, Amsterdam - London - Paris

16. GRABAR, P. & BURTIN, P. (1953), Biochim. Biophys. Acta 17, 67

17. SCHEIDEGGER, J. J. (1955), Int. Arch. Allergy 7, 103

18. CLAUSEN, J. & HEREMANS, J. (1960), J. Immunol. 84, 128

19. GRABAR, P. , Personal communication.

20. FRIEDRICH, F. W. (1971), Isolierung funktioneller Antikörper aus Rattenserum mit Hilfe der Methode der Immunadsorption und Darstellung monospezifischer Antiseren gegen die Immunglobuline der Ratte, Inauguraldissertation, Köln

21. HERMANN, G. , Unpublished

22. HEREMANS, J. F. (1960), Les Globulines Seriques du Systeme Gamma, Arscia, Bruxelles, and Masson, Paris

23. TALAL, N. , HERMANN, G. , De VAUX ST. , CYR, Ch. & GRABAR, P. (1964), J. Immunol. 92, 747

24. POTTER, M. & BOYCE, C. R. (1962), Nature (London) 193, 1086

25. DERNBACH, R. (1973), Das Verhalten von hämolysinbildenden Immunocyten bei Versuchen zur Induktion von Plasmosarkomen mit Bayol F bei der Ratte, Inauguraldissertation, Köln

26. FANTINI, F. , CATTANEO, R. & INVERNIZZI, F. (1967), Rheumatismo 19, 379

27. BAZIN,H.,DECKERS,C.,BECKERS,A. & HEREMANS,J.F. (1972), Int.J.Cancer 10, 568

28. QUERINJEAN,P.,BAZIN,H.,BECKERS,A.,DECKERS,C., HEREMANS,J.F. & MILSTEIN,C. (1972), Europ.J.Biochem. 31, 354

29. BAZIN,H.,BECKERS,A., BURTONBOY,G.,QUERINJEAN,P., MORIAME,M.,DECKERS,C. & HEREMANS,J.F. (1973), Ann.Imunol. Inst.Pasteur 124 C, 155

30. BAZIN,H.,BECKERS,A.,DECKERS,C. & MORIAME,M. (1973), J.Nat.Cancer Inst. 51, 1353

31. BAZIN,H.,BECKERS,A.,PLATTEAU,B.,DE METS,J. & KINTS,J.P.(1973), Exp.Animale 6, 219

32. BURTONBOY,G.,BAZIN,H.,DECKERS,C.,BECKERS,A., LAMY,M.E. & HEREMANS,J.F.(1973), Europ.J.Cancer 9, 259

33. BAZIN,H. (1974), Ann.Immunol. (Inst.Pasteur) 125 C, 277

34. BAZIN,H., BECKERS,A. & QUERINJEAN,P. (1974), Europ. J.Immunol. 4, 44

35. BAZIN,H.,BECKERS,A.,VAERMAN,J.P. & HEREMANS,J.F. (1974), J.Immunol. 112, 1035

36. BAZIN,H.,QUERINJEAN,P.,BECKERS,A.,HEREMANS,J.F. & DESSY,F. (1974), Immunology 26, 713

37. BECKERS,A.,QUERINJEAN,P. & BAZIN,H. (1974), Immuno-chemistry 11, 605

38. QUERINJEAN,P.,BAZIN,H.,KEHOE,J.M. & CAPRA,J.D. (1975), J.Immunol. 114, 1375

5.2 Immunological Differentiation of Monoclonal Immunoglobulins

H. Götz

Introduction

Monoclonal immunoglobulins, formerly called "paraproteins",
are homogeneous immunoglobulins produced by single clones of
B-dependent [1] plasma cells. Such appears to be the case in
certain malignant proliferative diseases of lymphocyte-like and
plasma cells usually associated with a high concentration of
related proteins in blood and other biological fluids. Such systemic processes are called "monoclonal gammopathies". In most
cases of such human diseases, as e. g. in myeloma, macro-
globulinemia WALDENSTRÖM and other lymphocyte and plasma cell disorders, only one clone is found proliferative.
Nevertheless, there are examples of malignant proliferations
not only of one but of two and even of three and more clones as
well (diclonal or triclonal gammopathies, respectively).

The homogeneous protein of monoclonal gammopathies may consist of complete molecules of one of the immunoglobulin classes
or subclasses, or of free light chains (Light Chain Disease,
BENCE-JONES Gammopathy), of free heavy chains (Heavy Chain
Disease, FRANKLIN's Disease) or of other forms of reduced or
degraded immunoglobulins, e. g. half molecules.

Monoclonal proteins generally lack antigen binding properties
although an increasing number of myeloma proteins has been
found in which antibody activity could be demonstrated.

---

1) B = Bursa equivalent

Principle Structure of Monoclonal Immunoglobulins

Based on pioneer work and on complete amino acid sequence analyses of human myeloma-, macroglobulin- and BENCE-JONES
proteins (1 - 11) the structure of monoclonal immunoglobulin
molecules may be briefly characterized as follows:

An immunoglobulin is comprised of two identical heavy chains
(molecular weight of each between 50 000 and 75 000) and two
identical light chains (molecular weight of each 22 500) which
are held together by disulfide bonds. This main structure is called "tetrapolypeptide" - or "four-chain polypeptide"-structure.
The nature of the heavy chains is representative for the individual
immunoglobulin classes, e. g. IgG, IgA, IgM, IgD and IgE, and
responsible for secondary biologic properties, such as complement fixation or cell attachment. The light chains are common to
all of the immunoglobulin classes, but a molecule of any class
may have two identical chains of either κ or λ . The quantitative relation between κ - and λ -chain molecules differs
from one immunoglobulin class to the other. Each polypeptide
chain is divided into a constant or C region and into a variable
or V region. The variable regions of heavy chains (V_H) and such
of light chains (V_L) include the identical antigen combining sites.
The various immunoglobulin classes differ characteristically in
the amino acid composition and sequence of their heavy chains,
in the number of their homology regions (domains) and to some
extent in size. Moreover, they differ in the number and location
of their interchain and intrachain disulfide bonds, in their con-
tents and position of oligosaccharides and the ability of polymerization.

The most important criterion of a monoclonal immunoglobulin is the fact, that it exists of a defined immunoglobulin class and of one type of light chains, only, e.g. either κ -chains or λ -chains.

Technical Aspects of Immunological Differentiation of Monoclonal Immunoglobulins

For the purpose of immunological characterization and differentiation of monoclonal proteins in patients' sera immunodiffusion techniques in gels or cellulose acetate foils offer a very useful adjunct in the diagnosis of malignant gammopathies.

Thanks to the widespread available polyspecific and monospecific antisera [2] against human serum and plasma proteins and against heavy and light chain properties of immunoglobulin classes an extensive analysis of serum samples may be undertaken in any laboratory.

The most important technique seems to be the immunoelectrophoresis (12, 13, 14, in 15). As it is known, this technique combines zonal electrophoresis with immunodiffusion including specific precipitin reactions between antigens (serum proteins) and homologous antibodies (in antisera). The resulting phenomena are visible arcs or bands of immunoprecipitate. Their electrophoretic position, their intensity and special shape dependent on

---

2) Antisera and antibody containing plates are commercially
   available, e.g. :
   Behringwerke AG, Marburg/Lahn (FRG),
   "medac" (Dacopatts), Hamburg (Danmark and FRG),
   Hyland/Travenol, München (USA and Munich),
   Miles-Serevac, Lausanne (Switzerland),
   Millipore, Neu-Isenburg (FRG),
   Celtec, Bad Homburg v. d. H. (FRG),
   Fresenius (Dr. E. Fresenius KG), Bad Homburg v. d. H. (FRG),
   Bio-Cult Laboratories, Berlin-West,
   Nordic Immunochemicals, Tilburg (Holland),
   Canalco Europe, Vlaadingen (Holland).

their immunoreaction with monospecific antisera are characteristic of their individual properties.

Other immunoelectrophoretic techniques, such as the twodimensional immunoelectrophoresis (16, 17) or the combined polyacryl-
amide- and agarose-immunoelectrophoresis (18, 19) are helpful
in special cases but not necessary for diagnostics in routine-
laboratories.

The twodimensional double immunodiffusion technique (20, in 15)
would be an additional method of detecting monoclonal immunoglobulins and of secundary antibody deficiency, but it is not equal
to immunoelectrophoresis.

In some cases it may be of clinical interest measuring the concentrations of monoclonal immunoglobulins in patients' sera over
a longer period. Here the indication is given of the single radial
immunodiffusion technique (21, in 15). It must be underlined, however, that this technique is acquainted with the possibility of a
certain failure: Using immunodiffusion plates with a defined concentration of monospecific antiserum, all homologous antigens,
e. g. monoclonal and polyclonal Ig-molecules are reacting with
the antibodies and give the precipitate the diameter of which is
measured for the quantitation.

Procedure of Analyses
Electrophoresis on cellulose acetate
Screen patients' sera with electrophoresis on cellulose acetate,
first of all! This is necessary for detection of monoclonal immunoglobulins concerning immunoglobulin classes such as IgD
or IgE. The antibody concentrations against IgD and IgE in polyspecific anti-human sera and even in monospecific anti-IgD and
anti- IgE are very low. In these cases it could be possible failing the typical precipitin arc because of the high antigen excess in
patients' sera.

For electrophoresis take a MICHAELIS buffer pH 8, 6, μ = 0,05.
Stain the stripes using Amidoschwarz 10 B.

Immunoelectrophoresis

In case of suspicion on a monoclonal gammopathy (see later),
screen the selected patients' sera with immunoelectrophoresis.
Concerning the supporting medium, agar gel, ionagar, agarose
gel and -stripes as well as cellulose acetate may be used in this
technique. The standard medium employed by the National Cancer
Institute's Immunoglobulin Reference Center, is agarose. Using
agar gel, the effect of electroendosmosis must be considered.

Take a 1, 2 perc. agar or agarose in MICHAELIS buffer pH 8, 6,
μ= 0, 05. The schematic arrangements of Figures 1 and 2 show
the major steps in the detection of monoclonal immunoglobulin
and the sequence which should be followed, using only one selected
serum (Fig. 1 and Fig. 2).

Take a glass plate (or cellulose- or agarose sheet) of 7, 5 by 9, 0
cm with seven channels for antisera and eight holes for the sera
examined, arranged as shown in Figures 1 and 2, cover the plates
with prepared agar or agarose gel, wait for the completion of
gelling and cut out the troughs and wells in the medium. For
electrophoresis take MICHAELIS buffer pH 8, 6, μ = 0, 05, 200 V
- 25 to 30 mA and 45 min per plate.

After having done immunoelectrophoresis in plate 1, take another
plate for detecting the type of L-chains or BENCE-JONES proteins, respectively (Fig. 2). According to the findings of plate 1
you may know the type of immunoglobulin class of the monoclonal
protein. Take the related monospecific antiserum of this immunoglobulin class for comparing the position of the κ - or λ -chain
in plate 2.

Biological Fluid: .... Date: ....
Patient's Name: ....
Address: .... IE Program: .....

Plate 1

Fig. 1

—————— N o —————— anti-HS (Human Serum, polyspecific)
—————— P o —————— anti-IgG
—————— N o —————— anti-IgA
—————— P o —————— anti-albumin or α_1 antitrypsin
—————— N o —————— anti-IgM
—————— P o —————— anti-IgD
—————— N o —————— anti-IgE
P o

Plate 2

Fig. 2

—————— N o 1 : 1 —————— anti-κ (BJ κ)
—————— P o 1 : 1 —————— anti-Ig (selected)
—————— N o 1 : 1 —————— anti-λ (BJ λ)
—————— P o 1 : 1 —————— anti-κ (BJ κ)
—————— P o 1 : 8 —————— anti-λ (BJ λ)
—————— P o 1 :16 —————— anti-κ (BJ κ)
—————— P o 1 : 24 —————— anti-λ (BJ λ)
P o 1 :32

N = Normal serum (reference serum)
P = Patient's serum
BJ = BENCE-JONES protein
IE = Immunoelectrophoresis (-phoretic)

Fig. 1 and 2. Schematic arrangements of immunoelectrophoretic analyses for the detection of monoclonal immuno-globulins.

As a quality control normal serum must be used on all plates for
reaction with each antiserum sample. Moreover, antisera employed must be compared with reference antisera.

If you elect to stain the plates wash and dry them before staining
with Amidoschwarz 10 B. Washing : Sodium chloride 0, 9 perc.
12 hours changing the bath four to five times. For a last bath take
distilled water. Drying: Under a filter paper at 37°C over night.
Staining: Amidoschwarz 10 B 1 g per liter in a solution of 500 ml
60 perc. acetic acid and 500 ml sodium acetate $\cdot$ 3 H_2O, 0,1 M.
Stain for one hour. Decolorize with a solution of 2 perc. acetic
acid in distilled water changing the bath up to a well decolorized
background. Add glycerol to a last bath in a concentration of about
1 perc. Allow plates to dry at room temperature.

Twodimensional double immunodiffusion technique
The indication of this technique is discussed above (p. 274). From
the practical point of view of the laboratorian or laboratory spe-
cialist it is not absolutely necessary.

Single radial immunodiffusion
The technique of single radial immunodiffusion in gels or sheets
of cellulose acetate and agarose dry preparations may be used for
the immunological quantitation of non monoclonal immunoglobulins
for diagnosis and observing the development of secundary antibody
deficiency. Additional, the technique is often achieved for measuring the concentrations of monoclonal immunoglobulins over a
longer period (see also p. 274).
Take purchasable antibody containing agar plates[2] and work as
indicated in the related instructions.

Electroimmunodiffusion technique

Alternatively to single radial immunodiffusion you may use the electroimmunodiffusion technique (22, 23) for measuring the concentrations of immunoglobulins. There are commercially available plates with monospecific antisera against IgG, IgA, and IgM [2]. Take them or prepare your own plates using agarose only (!) and work as indicated in the instructions.

Interpretation of the Results Obtained by Immunoelectrophoresis

Before reading the immunoelectrophoretic patterns look at the stained foils of cellulose acetate electrophoresis ! Monoclonal immunoglobulins may be already detected by a small peak within the protein fractions of a patient's serum. Such a peak must not only occur in a position where gamma globulins would be expected but may also appear (sometimes extremely) displaced from the gamma or beta globulin zone, e.g. from the α_1 to the post γ -globulin region.

As to immunoelectrophoretic findings, in normal sera the position of precipitin lines of the main immunoglobulin classes IgG, IgA and IgM is a very characteristic one and the shapes are consistent as long as the same procedure conditions are maintained (Fig. 3).

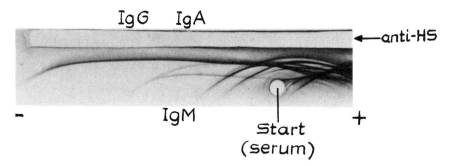

Fig. 3. Immunoelectrophoretic pattern of a normal serum -
Zone of immunoglobulins.

The IgG arc is the most prominent line of the slow migrating end of the human serum pattern. It is extremely elongated, from the $ß_1$ zone - sometimes even from the $α_1$ zone (!) - to the very end of the protein pattern.

IgA is characterized by a shorter and relatively faster running arc than IgG line and by a hook on its slow migrating end.

IgM is located high above the antibody trough and shows a straight and short line.

Any deviation in the shape or position of immunoglobulin arcs from that obtained by normal immunoglobulins developed under identical conditions indicates the existence of a monoclonal im-munoglobulin. Other abnormalities are indicated by an obvious decrease or the complete absence of precipitin lines characteris-tic for non monoclonal immunoglobulins as described above. More-over, monoclonal immunoglobulins can often be detected by a displacement and by the phenomenon of an antigen excess, e.g. broadening of the precipitin band.

Using polyspecific anti-human antisera, in most cases it seems to be sufficient analyzing the pathologic serum in normal concen-tration only (Fig. 4). For identifying the L-type, however, it is necessary testing the patient's serum in several dilutions (see Fig. 2, Fig. 5). This is implied by the antigen excess in most of the monoclonal gammopathies and by the low concentrations of antibodies against L-chain types found in nearly all commercially available L-chain antisera.

In samples of IgG myeloma precipitin phenomena are seen indi-cating the existence of a monoclonal (or diclonal) immunoglobulin and "normal", that means polyclonal IgG molecules, too (see Fig. 4). Deviations of the IgG line may be found in regions from the fast migrating $α_1$-globulins to $γ$-globulins migrating slower than "physiological" immunoglobulins of class G.

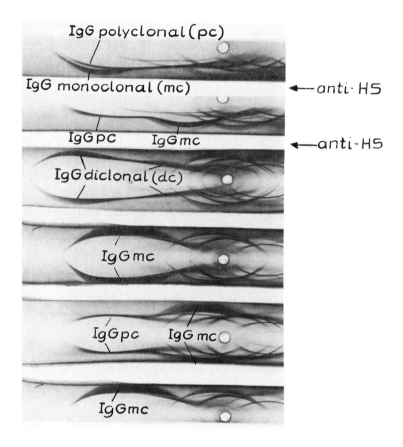

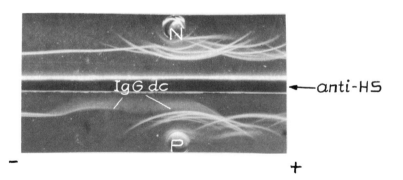

Fig. 4. Immunoelectrophoretic patterns of different IgG
myeloma sera examined undiluted and precipitated by
polyspecific anti-human serum (Hyland Laboratories/
Travenol International, Munich).

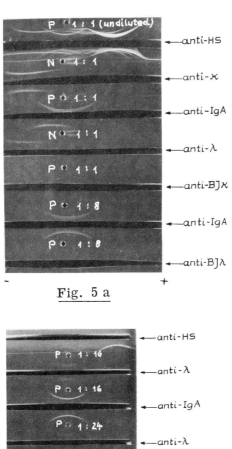

Fig. 5 a

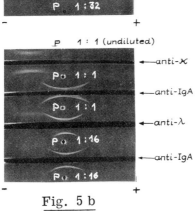

Fig. 5 b

Fig. 5 a , b. Immunoelectrophoretic plates with analyses of an
IgA myeloma serum.
Antisera in Fig. 5a and 5b above: Behringwerke AG,
Marburg/Lahn; Antisera in Fig. 5b below: Medac,
Hamburg.

In cases of <u>IgA myeloma</u> displacements from the position of α_1-
to that of fast migrating IgG can be detected. Such "electrophoretic polymorphisms" may perhaps be dependent on the ability of
forming polymers by IgA. Pay attention to the α-zone because
of a relative frequent appearance of monoclonal IgA in this region
(so-called α-paraproteins)! IgA and also monoclonal IgA tends to
form complexes with non-immunoglobulins, e.g. albumin or α_1-
antitrypsin (24, 25, 26) probably by a function of J-chains (26, 27).[3]
Thus, the immunological identification of such reactions makes
the diagnosis of monoclonal IgA quite sure (Fig. 6).

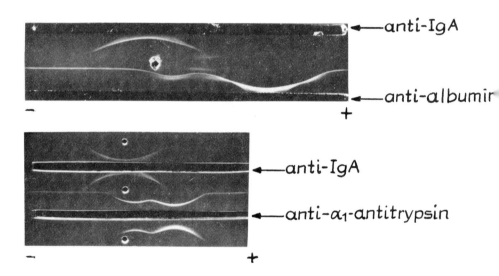

Fig. 6. Demonstration of complexes formed between IgA and
albumin and IgA and α_1 antitrypsin as well. Immunoelectrophoresis of the same serum as in Fig. 5a, b.

[3] Not only IgA myelomas are forming complexes with non-immunoglobulins - there are observations of binding activities between IgG
myeloma protein and α_2-macroglobulin, IgG and lysozyme, IgM
macroglobulin and albumin, IgG and transferrin, IgG and ß-lipoprote-
in and even between free L -chains and pre-albumin and/or α_1-
antitrypsin - but IgA myeloma proteins show in most of the cases
examined complex forming abilities as discussed (including own
experience).

Monoclonal IgM shows various types of precipitin phenomena:
Elongation of the line with a "butcher's hook" at the slow migrating end, occurrence of two or three bulges with the criterion of
immunologic identity reaction, shortening and thickening of the
arc or presence of a very dense precipitate close to the antigen
well in the absence of the normal IgM line.

For the detection of monoclonal IgD and IgE it would be of urgen-
cy using a series of diluted serum samples already in the first
plate of immunoelectrophoretic analysis.

IgD myeloma proteins have the tendency to degrade (or depoly-
merize ?). Thus, the IgD of one and the same myeloma serum
may appear once in the β_1 region and, after a period of staying
at $+ 4^{O}C$ perhaps in the zone of α-globulins. The precipitin arc
often forms a bow from α_1- to β_1-globulins in such cases (Fig. 7).

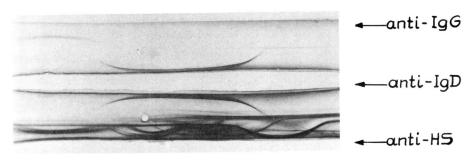

←—anti-IgG

←—anti-IgD

←—anti-HS

Fig. 7. A special case of IgD myeloma. Immunoelectrophoretic
pattern.

Myeloma globulins of class IgE have been described by three
different authors (28, 29, 30), only.*)

BENCE-JONES gammopathy is diagnosed by the detection exclu-
sively of light chains, either type κ or type λ, without any indication of the existence of heavy chains. Thanks to the fact that
light chains appear in the patient's urine the identification in that
biological fluid proves successful in most of the cases.

*) The communication of a fourth case is given by STOICA, G.H., but not yet
published.

<u>Heavy Chain Disease</u> is detected by finding only H-chains (mostly Fc fragment) of a defined immunoglobulin class using monospecific antisera against γ-, α-, μ-, δ- and ϵ-properties. Before confirming the diagnosis of such a relatively seldom disorder, any examinations with the serum sample (long series of dilutions !) must be undertaken to exclude the existence of light chains. H-chains may be found in serum and urine.

With regard to the <u>abundance ratio</u> of the different classes of monoclonal immunoglobulins it seems to be obvious that it is in accordance with the quantitative relations of polyclonal immuno-globulins of man. That means, that IgG gammopathies represent the most cases of detected monoclonal immunoglobulins whereas IgE myelomas occur as the fewest ones.

Concerning the <u>development</u> of multiple myeloma, macroglobu-linemia WALDENSTRÖM and related diseases, the pathogenetic factors seem to be the same ones as such in cases of malignant tumors and proliferative disorders of the "reticulo-histiocytic system". Thus, in myeloma plasma cells have been found with "new" membrane antigens comparable with tumor-specific sur-face antigens. The special ability of B-dependent immunocom-petent cells to deliver complete or deficient immunoglobulins facilitate the clinical diagnosis in such cases.

Summary

The present paper deals with the immunological differentiation of monoclonal immunoglobulins. In a short preface the principle structure of monoclonal immunoglobulins is pointed out. In the main part of this communication, technical aspects as well as interpretation remarks on immunological, especially immuno-electrophoretic findings of patients' sera are submitted and discussed.

Acknowledgement: The immunoelectrophoretic and other immunological analyses performed in our research laboratory were carried out with the assistance of Mrs. I. ANDERS. I wish to thank
her for excellent collaboration.

References

1. DEUTSCH, H. F. & MORTON, J. I. (1957), Science 125, 600

2. PORTER, R. R. (1959), Biochem. J. 73, 119

3. EDELMAN, G. M. & POULIK, M. D. (1961), J. Exp. Med. 113, 861

4. PUTNAM, F. W. , EASY, C. W. & LYNN, L. T. (1962), Biochim.
    Biophys. Acta 58, 279

5. FLEISCHMAN, J. B., PORTER, R. R. & PRESS, E. M. (1963),
    Biochem. J. 88, 220

6. EDELMAN, G. M. & GALLY, J. A. (1964), Proc. Nat. Acad.
    Sci. USA 51, 846

7. HILSCHMANN, N. & CRAIG, L. C. (1965), Proc. Nat. Acad.
    Sci. USA 53, 1403

8. HILSCHMANN, N. (1967), Hoppe-Seyler's Z. Physiol. Chem.
    348, 1077

9. HILSCHMANN, N. (1969), Naturwissenschaften 56, 195

10. HILSCHMANN, N. , PONSTINGL, H. , WATANABE, S. ,
    BARNIKOL, H. U. , BACZKO, K. , BRAUN, M. & LEIBOLD,
    W. (1972), FEBS Sympos. 26, 31

11. PUTNAM, F. W. (1974), Progr. Immunology II, vol. 1, p. 25
    (eds. Brent, L. and Holborow, J.) North-Holland Publishing
    Company, Amsterdam - Oxford. American Elsevier Publish-
    ing Company, Inc. , New York

12. GRABAR, P. & WILLIAMS, C. A. (1953), Biochim. Biophys.
    Acta 10, 193

13. GRABAR, P. & BURTIN, P. (1964), Immunelektrophoretische
    Analyse, Elsevier Publishing Company, Amsterdam

14. SCHEIDEGGER, J. J. (1955), Int. Arch. Allergy 7, 103

15. GÖTZ, H. (1973), Immunologische Plasmaprotein-Diagnostik,
    Walter de Gruyter & Co. , Berlin - New York

16. LAURELL, C. B. (1965), Anal. Biochem. 10, 358

17. CLARKE, M. H. G. & FREEMAN, T. (1968), Clin. Sci. 35, 403

18. BIEL, H. & ZWISLER, O. (1966), Behringwerk-Mitteilungen 46, 141

19. ZWISLER, O. & BIEL, H. (1966), Behringwerk-Mitteilungen 46, 129

20. OUCHTERLONY, Ö. (1949), Acta Pathol. Microbiol. Scand. 26, 507

21. MANCINI, G. , CARBONARA, A. & HEREMANS, J. F. (1965), Immunochemistry 2, 235

22. LAURELL, C. B. (1966), Anal. Biochem. 15, 45

23. LAURELL, C. B. (1972), Scand. J. Clin. Lab. Invest. 29, Suppl. 124, 21

24. HEREMANS, J. F. (1960), Les Globulines Sériques du Système Gamma. Leur Nature et leur Pathologie, Arscia, Bruxelles and Masson, Paris

25. MANNIK, M. (1967), J. Immunol. 99, 899

26. HEREMANS, J. F. (1974), Behring Institute - Mitteilungen 54, 1

27. TOMASI, T. B. (1973), Ref. International Symposium on Immunoglobulin A System, Birmingham, Alabama, Oct. 23 - 25, Plenum Press, New York

28. JOHANSSON, S. G. O. & BENNICH, H. (1967), in Gamma Globulins (ed. Killander, J.) Nobel Symposium 3, p. 193, Almqvist & Wiksell, Stockholm

29. OGAWA, M. , KOCHWA, S. , SMITH, C. , ISHIZAKA, K. & McINTYRE, O. R. (1969), N. Engl. J. Med. 281, 1217

30. FISHKIN, B. G. , ORLOFF, N. , SCADUTO, L. E. , BORUCKI, D. T. & SPIEGELBERG, H. L. (1972), Blood 39, 361

5.3 Lung Neoplasia and Paraproteinemia

C. Ricci, C. Baldi and R. Bonardi

There are principally two types of paraproteinaemia not correlated with myeloma, WALDENSTRÖM's macroglobulinaemia and
lymphoma.

These are the so-called, "idiopathic paraproteinaemias with no
clinical implications"[1,2], in which the M component was only
found during a protein screening, because of an increased erythrocytes'sedimentation value.

In the second group, there are symptomatic conditions which may
be present in malignant diseases and less frequently in autoimmune conditions [1,3].

From a nosologic point of view we should include symptomatic
paraproteinaemias in immunoproliferative diseases following the
suggestions of DAMESHEK [4] and MARMONT et al.[5].

A modern cellular subgrouping of immunoproliferative disease
could be the following one:

Abnormal Plasmacellular Proliferation
Multiple myeloma
Mixed cryoglobulinaemia
Heavy chain disease [FRANKLIN's disease]
Symptomatic and idiopathic paraproteinaemia
Abnormal Lymphocyte Proliferation
WALDENSTRÖM's macroglobulinaemia
Chronic lymphatic leukaemia

Cold agglutinin disease

Heavy chain disease [FRANKLIN's disease]

Lymphosarcoma with paraproteinaemia

Abnormal Reticular Proliferation

Reticular sarcoma [there are only single rare forms with para-
proteinaemias].

Following the concept expressed by BELLANTI [6], monoclonal immunoglobulins could be the end result of extreme clonal stimulation by an abnormal antigenic agent.

Monoclonal immunoglobulin components have frequently been discovered in the serum of patients suffering from a variety of neoplastic diseases other than malignancies of immunoglobulin-producing cell types [3,7].

Such associations appear to be rather frequent, since malignancies were discovered in 31 of OSSERMANN and TAKATSUK's [8] 400 cases with M components, 10 of RIVA's 33 [1] cases and 29 of HÄLLEN's [9] 138 cases.

There is no proof of paraprotein production by epithelial cells belonging to malignant proliferation of the lungs; on the other hand, the rich accumulation of immunocompetent cells in the submucosal tract of the bronchial tree should be stressed. These cells produce IgA as well as IgE immunoglobulins following antigenic stimulation. A shift is also possible in the production of the immunoglobulin type.

In addition to the view that a monoclonal immunoglobulin disorder and cancer in a patient is an accidental occurrence, several alternative explanations have been proposed. Among these are:

a] The possibility of the conditions having the same underlying basis, a congenital or inherited defect, exposure to a common carcinogenic, chemical, viral agent.

b] The monoclonal immunoglobulin might arise in response to the cancer, either as the result of antigenic stimulation or direct pro- duction by cell types which do not normally produce immunoglo- bulins.

c] The presence of a monoclonal immunoglobulin disorder might signify an abnormality of cell mediated immunity causing failure of the immunologic monitoring system to remove mutant cells and also permitting the emergence of one or more antibody–producing monoclones of immunocytes.

Recently we had occasion to observe some cases of association between lung cancer and paraproteinaemia.

We should briefly like to present the following three cases.

Methods

Protein studies were made following acrylamide gel electro- phoresis, immunoelectrophoresis, following the micromethod of SCHEIDEGGER [11], immunodiffusion with anti-light chain an- tisera, following the techniques of BARANDUN et al.[12], quan- titative immunodiffusion techniques following the MANCINI et al. [13] technique. Haematological, serological and histological studies were carried out following the routine investigation pro- cedure.

First case

Mario R., born at Como 27/7/11.

Family history: no familial or hereditary disease.

Physiological history: heavy drinker [1 - 1 1/2 litre/day]; 15-20 cigarettes per day.

Pathological history: hospitalized 1959 and 1960 for fever episodes diagnosed as bronchopulmonitis. Admitted for left subclavicular fibro-ulcerous condition lasting two months in 1965. Winter episodes of coughing with sputum since the age of 40. Admitted for sudden high fever, persistent cough and deterioration of general conditions in 1969.

Objective examination: poorly nourished subject.

Respiratory apparatus: expanded chest, with reduced elasticity; widespread hyperphonesis with lowered, hypokinetic bases; marked bronchial breathing, with diffused rhonchi and rales.

Left upper lobe; further reduction of alveolar breathing, coupled with subcrepitant rales. Slight increase in liver size [2 cm from arch] and consistency.

Laboratory data ESR 116 mm/1st hr. RCC 3,400,000; Hb 12.2 g/100 ml; WCC 7,500 [N 75, E 1, B 1, L 22, M 1]; MCV 110; MCHC 31%. Urine: negative. All other biochemical data within the limits of normal.

Sputum negative for KOCH bacillus. Proteins 8,2 g/100 ml.
Cellulose acetate electrophoresis: α_1-globulins 4.0%; α_2-globulins 13.0%; β_1-globulins 5.5%; β_2 globulins and γ-globulins, 40.5%. Albumin-globulin ratio: 0.59 [monoclonal peak in the β - γ position].

Chest X-ray: bronchopulmonic involvement of the right upper lobe, together with increased, chronic bronchitic type density, fibrosis attributable to prior episodes, and notable emphysema.

Hospitalization lasted 28 days on this occasion. Penycillin, tetracycline and cephalosporine were administered, coupled with prophylactic isoniazide. The patient's general condition improved considerably. A similar improvement was noted in the respira-

tory picture, including complete reabsorption of bronchopneumon-
ic foci. Signs of inflammation diminished. ESR was 68 mm/ 1 st
hr. Monoclonal hypergammaglobulinaemia persisted.

The patient was readmitted with asthenia, slight fever, anorexia,
persistent cough and loss of weight on 26/2/71. A marked deterioration in general condition was noted on objective examination.
Loss of vocal fremitus in the left apical and scapular area, with
increased density on percussion. Breathing appeared to be shal-
lower on this side.

Apical respiratory silence; murmuring respiration, with low-
frequency expiration noise at the lingular segments. Signs of
widespread emphysematous bronchitis were also observed.

Hepatomegaly [2 cm from the arch] was again noted, as in 1969.
Evidence of peripheral polyneuropathy [bilateral loss of ACHILLES
reflex] was also obtained.

Standard chest radiography showed extensive opaqueness of the
upper lung field and left hiloparahilar area, with slight displacement of the cardiovascular shadow and upward movement of the
left hemidiaphragm. Stratigraphy revealed increased left hiloparahilar density, with engulfment of the upper lobar bronchus and
atelectasis of the dependent parenchyma. Marked coarctation of
the lingular bronchus with ectasia of the post-stenotic tract.

The sputum was mucous and GRAM-positive cocci predominated
in its bacterial flora. KOCH bacillus was absent. Few epithelial
cells and leukocytes were noted though there were some neoplastic cells. S. pyogenes, NEISSERIAE and KLEBSIELLAE were
cultured.

Blood picture: Hb 15 g; RCC 5,000,000; WCC 8,500 [N 65, E 2, B 0, M 1, L 32]. ESR 70 mm/1st hr. Normal blood urea, sugar, uric acid, lipids, Na, K and Ca.

Acrylamide gel electrophoresis: proteins 7·9 g/100 ml; albumins 30.5; α_1-globulins 4.0; α_2-globulins 5.5; ß1-globulins 6.0; ß$_2$-globulins 5.5; γ_1-globulins 29·5; γ_2-globulins 9·0. Monoclonal peak in the ß - γ position.
No significant changes noted in three further examinations in the following months. Immunoelectrophoresis pointed to the presence of an IgG K paraprotein.

Immunodiffusion: IgA 396 mg/100 ml; IgM 88 mg/100 ml; IgG over 5000 mg/100 ml.

Urinary protein values were not pathological and **BENCE JONES** proteins were not observed.

No radiological signs of osteolysis [cranium spine, pelvis, ribs]. Blood calcium was always below 10 mg/100 ml. Marrow biopsy: normal red and white cells with a small number of megakaryocytes. Plasma cells: 30% with no morphological changes worthy of note.

Bronchoscopy: concave stop in the left upper lobar bronchus. No neoplastic cells in the aspirated material. Bronchography: confirmation of stop, with amputation of the dorsal and anterior apical branches. By contrast, the lingular bronchus presented smooth-edged stenosis at its origin, followed by cylindrical ecstatic dilatation. Lung scintiscan: [99 Tc-labelled albumin microspheres]: serious reduction of flow over the entire left lung, with amputation of the upper lobe vessels.

BSF test: diminished clearance [approx. 30% retention at 45"].

Normal blood bilirubin and transaminases. Liver scintiscan [colloidal ^{198} Au]: slight hepatopsis, size within normal limits. Marked reduction of overall granulopexic capacity, with incipient activation of the splenic histiocyte reticulum.

Urea clearance: slight reduction of glomerular filtrate. Radiography of the digestive tract: imbutiform restriction of the antrum, with slight asymmetry and rigidity of the walls. Altered loading of the greater curvature was interpreted as scleroatrophic gastritis with perivisceritis.

Final diagnosis: malignant neoplasia of the left superior lobar bronchus, with hilar metastasis. Chronic emphysematous bronchitis. Sequels of left subclavicular TB. Scleroatrophic gastritis. Concomitant IgG K paraproteinaemia.

Clinical course: following continuous hospitalization lasting almost three months, the patient died as a result of an episode of cardiocirculatory insufficiency on 16/2/72.

Necropsy: acute plurivisceral stasis. Pulmonary and cerebral aedema. Dilatation of the cardiac cavities. Hypertrophy of the ventricles. Myocardial brown atrophy and sclerosis. Bronchogenic squamous carcinoma of the left upper lobe, with hilar lymphnode metastases. Bullous emphysema of the right lung. Bilateral pleural fibro-adhesions. Ulcerated cystopapilliferous gastric carcinoma. Perisplenitis.

Second case

Giuseppe C., mechanic, born at Saronno [Varese] on 29/9/1920. Family history: negative. Physiological history: moderate smoker [10-15 per day].

Pathological history: first admitted Saronno hospital [23/2/66], for ulcerated gingival swelling on left mandible [678], together with general malaise, anorexia and slight fever. A local biopsy showed inflammation with caseous granulomas of certain TB origin.

Chest X-ray: bilateral miliary infiltration. Considerable infiltration and multi-excavation in both apexes. Left pleural apico-axillary thickening, with hilipetous fibrotic striae.

Emergency sanatorium treatment was followed by discharge as clinically cured after about 30 days, with a recommendation to present for out-patient controls.

The patient enjoyed good health until a few weeks prior to a second period of hospitalization starting 3/3/72. On this occasion, the initial picture included burning, abscess-type pain over the whole of the left half of the chest, with persistent cough, little sputum and effort dyspnoea.

Objective examination: signs of chronic bronchitis and emphysema [expanded chest, tympanic hyperphonesis, lowered and poorly mobile bases, widespread bronchiolised breathing], with a vast area [corresponding to the projection of the left upper lobe] frankly dense on percussion and practically devoid of respiratory activity.

Chest-X-ray: massive, roundish opaqueness in the middle left anterior field, with adenopathic enlargement of the hilus and downward displacement of the trachea. Sequels of diaphragmatic pachypleuritis.

Blood picture: Hb 13.4 g/100 ml; RCC 5,100,000; WCC 7,300 [N 65, B 1, E 1, L 31, M 1]; MCV 82; MCHC 31; ESR 118 mm/1st hr. Normal blood uric acid, sugar, urea, Na and K.

Cellulose acetate electrophoresis:

	4/2/72	7/3/72
Proteins	7.95	7.1
Albumins	34.0	41.0
α_1-globulins	4.0	3.5
α_2-globulins	13.0	11.5
β_1-globulins	7.0	8.5
β_2-globulins	5.5	5.5
γ_1-globulins	1.15	13.0
γ_2-globulins	21.5	17.0

Immunodiffusion: IgA 224 mg/100 ml; IgM 66 mg/100 ml; IgG 3270 mg/100 ml. Immunoelectrophoresis:IgG K paraprotein. Blood calcium: less than 10 mg/100 ml. Normal acid and alkaline phosphatase. Normal bone X-ray. No aspecific or BENCE JONES urinary proteins.

Marrow biopsy: rich in both white and red cells, especially the former; normal white cell maturation. Increased plasma cells [50%].

Bronchography: penetration of the main left lobe proved impossible with a straight catheter. A gravity-administered contrast medium showed downward and rightward compression deformation of the main bronchus and trachea, caused by well-defined mediastinal masses. The upper lobe bronchi were frankly distorted and interrupted after a short distance by the rat-tailed lobar branch of the anterior segmentary lobe. The lingular branches were amputated at their origin.

Stratigraphy confirmed the presence of large neoplastic masses in the middle field and anterior lingular segment, together with hilar and paratracheal masses of probable metastatic origin.

Lung scintiscan [^{51}Cr-labeled albumin microspheres]:seriously reduced uptake in the left upper lobe, indicating pronounced alteration of the parenchymal flow.

Final diagnosis: neoplasia of the left upper lobe, with hilar and mediastinal metastasis in a subject with chronic bronchitis and pulmonary emphysema, fibrosclerosis from TB and concomitant paraproteinaemia.

Clinical course: The patient received a single i.v. dose of 2 g cyclophosphamide, followed by scalar 45 mg/day prednisone. Further hospitalization due to worsening of the clinical picture was required on 5/4/72, 26/7/72, and 4/9/72.

There was marked general and, more particularly, respiratory ingravescence on these occasions. Swelling of the soft parts in the left subclavicular area due to parietal infiltration was also observed. Episodes of serious respiratory insufficiency and pulmonary oedema occurred during the last two periods, with a terminal picture of irreversible shock. The patient was discharged at the relatives' request and no necropsy was performed.

It may be noted that administration of a total of 6 g i.v. cyclophosphamide was followed by a marked improvement in the electrophoretic protein picture [see attached trace].

Third case

Sergio M., aged 41 years, mechanic.

Family history: no familial or hereditary diseases.

Physiological history: heavy smoker[40 per day] and drinker [1 - 1 1/2 litres per day].

Pathological history: excellent health until February 1971, when a chest X-ray carried out on account of asthenia, indefinite joint pains and loss of weight showed roundish opaque patches of varying size up to the diameter of a plum on the right upper lobe. Out patient control till November 1971 was followed by hospitalization for right supramammary and subscapular pain. The progressive course of the disease was made clear on this occasion in the form of multiple opaque patches, some of them transient, on both sides. A single dose of cyclophosphamide produced marked pulmonary remission [diminished opacity] and an improvement in general condition. Regression of HIPPOCRATES fingers was also observed.

Continued evolution of the clinical picture led to a further period of hospitalization for bronchological examination. The objective picture was one of poor general condition, normal pressure, dyspnoea and marked HIPPOCRATES fingers.

Chest picture: slight hypophonesis in both bases, weak vocal fremitus, vesicular murmur, no rhonchi or rales. X-ray: secondary nodules scattered over both lungs. The largest [about the size of a plum] extended as far as a right interclavicularhilar site and had a non-uniform shadow tone.

Blood picture: Hb 91.3 g/100 ml, RCC 4,680,000; WCC 8,900 [N 71, E 2, B 0, M 1, L 26]. ESR [Kata] 9.
Total proteins: 7.9 g/100 ml. Acrylamide gel electrophoresis: albumins 54; α_1-globulins 3; α_2-globulins 13; β_1-globulins 20; γ_2 globulins 10. Monoclonal peak in the γ_1-position.
Immunodiffusion: [BARANDUN's double line technique] using an anti-light-chain antiserum showed monoclonal IgG K; this was confirmed by electrophoresis.
TB and Aspergillus fumigatus skin reaction: negative.

The bronchoscopy picture was normal. Two bronchial washings for PAPANICOLAU cell study were carried out. The first showed [inter alia]: small group of pavement cells, with little cytoplasm and large hyperchromic nuclei. Similar cells were also observed in small quantities of granulofilamentous material in the sediment, together with a small strip of pavement epithelium on several rows of cells with dissimilar nuclei, some pyknotic and some hyperchromic. These findings were not considered sufficient for positive diagnosis and class I assessment.

On the second occasion; however, this classification was strongly supported by a finding of numerous lymphocytes, histiocytes, granulocytes and superficial pavement epithelium cells; columnar cells were much less in evidence. Epithelial cells with little cytoplasm and large, distinctly hyperchromic nuclei were occasionally observed. The sediment gave the same picture.

Standard methods and electrophoresis following ultrafiltration showed an absence of BENCE JONES urinary proteins. Further examination was prevented by the patient's voluntary discharge.

Conclusions

These three cases of lung cancer ran a particularly rapid course. Death occurred within 3 and 8 months from admission for observation in cases 1 and 2. The third patient died within one year and presented marked signs of dissemination when he left hospital. The clinical picture was dominated by local physiopathological lung alterations, with terminal cardiorespiratory insufficiency. Apart from a fleeting response in the third case, treatment was without effect. Diagnosis was both histological and cytological on all occasions. Necropsy revealed secondary and minor gastric cystopapilliferous carcinoma in the first case. Paraproteinaemia was noted during close serum examination. It was, however, always of secondary importance and unaccompanied by clinical signs, particularly the skeletal involvement typical of malignant lymphocyte and plasma cell proliferation. It was, in fact, an example of paraneoplastic paraproteinsaemia.

Idiopathic and secondary paraproteinaemias are recognized, covering clinical pictures of neoplasia involving various sites, within the general classification of immunoproliferative disease. The physiopathological and etiopathogenetic importance of a finding of this kind is not entirely clear.

The view that proliferation of primarily epithelial neoplastic cells might be accompanied by the production of pathological immuno-globulins has been abandoned since WILLIAMS's [14] immuno-fluorescent studies showed that these cells were non-secretive. It has also been shown that the cells responsible for such pro-duction may be immunocytes surrounding the neoplasia. These studies were directed to cancer of the colon. It may be recalled that the submucosa of the large intestine is particularly rich in plasmolymphocytes and that these are mainly secretors of "secretory" IgA's.

Applications of these findings to the case of the lungs find an echo in a similar richness in the submucosa of the entire bron-chial tree. In this case, the cells are concerned with the secre-tion of immunoglobulins for both cell and humoral defence against antigens.

In the opinion of BELLANTI [6] paraproteins can be seen as a self-perpetuating response to prolonged antigen stimulus.

By way of hypothesis, it may be supposed that, whereas the oc-currence of autoimmunological phenomena constitutes the first response to a tumor antigen, a papaprotein is the last, and unfortunately the least effective, response of the same kind. From the conceptual standpoint, the observation of paraproteins in the three cases reported here is attached to the question of possible antibody activity on the part of monoclonal proteins. This question was not considered in the present study. A paper by RIVA [15], however, has given further proof of the frequent antibody activity noted in the so-called idiopathic and secondary paraproteinaemias.

Closer examination of this point might be of interest in assessing the significance of the observation of a paraneoplastic monoclonal gamma globulin.

References

1. RIVA, G.[1964], Helvet.Med.Acta 31, 285

2. DESPONT,J.P.,FLUCKIGER,R.,GRAITH,A.,HAUSSER, E.,JEANNET,M.,MONNIER,J.,SCHEIDEGGER,J.J., SIEGENTHALER,P.,WETTSTEIN,P.& CRUCHAUD,A. [1969],Helvet.Med.Acta 34, 401

3. MICHAUX,J.L.,& HEREMANS,J.F.[1969],Amer.J.Med. 46, 562

4. DAMESHEK,W.[1970], The Immunoproliferative Disorders in Regulation of Hematopoisis [ed.Gordon,S.] Appleton-Century-Crofts,New York

5. MARMONT,A. & DAMASIO,E.[1972],Rec.Progr.Med.53, 2

6. BELLANTI,A. [1971],Immunology,W.B.Saunders Company, Philadelphia - London -Toronto

7. HOBBS,J.R.[1971],Immunoglobulins in clinical chemistry, in Advances in Clinical Chemistry,vol. 14,Academic Press, New York - London

8. OSSERMAN,E.F.& TAKATSUKI,K.[1963],Medicine 42, 357

9. HÄLLEN,J.[1966],Acta Med.Scand. 179[Suppl.462], 1

10. ZAWADZKI,Z.A. & EDWARDS,G.[1972],Non myelomatous monoclonal immunoglobulinemia, in Progress in Immunology, vol. 1, Grune & Stratton,New York - London

11. SCHEIDEGGER, J. J. [1955], Int. Arch. Allergy 7, 103

12. BARANDUN, S., CARREL, S., GERBER, H., MORELL, A., RIESEN, W. & SKVARIL, F. [1971], Schweiz. Med. Wochenschr. 101, 955

13. MANCINI, G., CARBONARA, A. O. & HEREMANS, J. F. [1965], Immunochemistry 2, 235

14. WILLIAMS, R. C. & HOWE, R. [1969], Amer. J. Med. Sci. 257, 275

15. RIVA, G. [1972], Le paraproteinemie idiopatiche e di accompagnamento. Relazione al Simposio Internazionale sulle Gammopatie monoclonali, Accademia dei Lincei, Roma.

6 Some Clinical Aspects

6.1 Lymphocyte Transformation in Malignant Diseases. Communication II: Results in Reticulo- and Lymphoproliferative Diseases as well as in Carcinomas

A. Pappas and P. G. Scheurlen

In the past few years, there have been many experimental and clinical observations indicating a close relationship between immunological reactions and malignant diseases [1-12]. The immunological system functions as a "surveillance" in that that transformed cells, which provoke specific, cell-mediated immune reactions in the organism, are rejected, and a malignant proliferation is thus prevented [13-18]. Disturbances of the immune system, such as prolonged treatment with immunosuppressive agents, lead to a significant increase in the appearance of malignant neoplasias [19]. The reduction in the cellular immune reaction in cases of malignant lymphoreticular diseases and other malignant tumors has long been recognized [20-22]. Lymphocytes, as mediators of the immune reaction, -T-lymphocytes primarily for the cellular and B-lymphocytes for the humoral immune reaction - play an important role in the host organism's resistance to malignant growth [8-10].

The transformation of the blood lymphocytes by phytohemagglutinin [PHA] in vitro serves as an indirect measure of the late type of immune reaction.

Materials and Methods

Using the previously described methods [23], we examined the transformability or the [^{14}C] thymidine incorporation of peripheral lymphocytes in the presence of PHA. The lymphocytes were taken from the following groups of patients:

1. 47 patients with lymphogranulomatosis [M. HODGKIN] in
    Stage I - II or III - IV. We used the clinical and pathological
    criteria given by PERRY [24] to determine the stage of the
    disease. According to this classification, 14 of the patients
    we examined were in Stage I-II at the time of the culturing,
    and 33 were in Stage III-IV. Except for two patients in Stage
    II and three in Stage III-IV, all of the patients had been pre-
    viously treated with corticosteroids and/or cytostatic agents.
    At the time of the experiments, 18 of the patients had received
    no chemical therapy in the preceeding six weeks. In eight
    patients the relative number of lymphocytes was in the nor-
    mal range, while a definite lymphopenia was present in the
    others.

2. Of 42 patients with chronic lymphatic leukemia, 20 had not
    yet been treated at the time the cells were taken for culture.
    In 21 cases, the disease had been present between 1 and 7
    years. One patient had suffered a chronic lymphatic leuke-
    mia for 15 years. In 14 cases, the leucocyte number was
    more than 50 000 leucocytes/mm^3, and in the other 28, the
    number was below 50 000/mm^3.

3. Blood lymphocytes from the following groups were cultivated
    with PHA and their [^{14}C] thymidine incorporation recorded:
    27 patients with stomach carcinoma, 13 patients with adeno-
    carcinoma of the stomach, and 26 patients with stomach or
    duodenal ulcers. The results were compared with those of
    50 healthy controls. The diagnoses were gastroscopically
    and histologically confirmed.

4. The effect of the plasma of the following 22 patients with
    malignant diseases on the transformation in vitro of lympho-
    cytes from healthy subjects was measured. The lymphocytes
    were stimulated with phytohemagglutinin and tuberculin [PPD].

Four lymphogranulomatoses, Stage IV, one HODGKIN sarcoma, one reticular sarcoma, one acute leukemia, two hyper-
nephromas, two portio carcinomas, one prostate carcinoma,
one colon carcinoma, one stomach carcinoma, one liver
carcinoma, two chronic myeloic leukemias, one chronic
lymphatic leukemia, three adenocarcinomas, and one tes-
ticular teratoma.

The plasma of three healthy persons served as a control.
The plasma was separated into 4 fractions on Sephadex
G-200 as described previously [23]. Fraction IV was then
rechromatographed on Sephadex G-25. The effects of whole
plasma and the separate fractions were tested. 2 ml of the
patient plasma or the chromatographically separated fraction
[reconcentrated to the original concentration] was added to
10 ml culture together with 150 μg PPD or 0.1 ml PHA.
Controls were run with autologous plasma. The incubation
time for PHA cultures was 3 days, and for PPD cultures,
5 days.

Results

1. Lymphogranulomatoses:

The transformation rate [% blast cells] and [^{3}H]- or [^{14}C] thymidine incorporation depended on the stage of the disease in a
total of 47 patients examined [Fig. 1 and 2]. The lymphocytes
of 14 patients in Stage I -II reacted almost normally after 72-
hour stimulation by PHA [Fig. 1 and 2].

The transformation and incorporation rates were independent
a] of the number of lymphocytes in the peripheral blood and
b] of the treatment. In all the lymphocyte cultures from 33 patients in Stage III - IV, the rates of transformation and [^{3}H]- or
[^{14}C] thymidine incorporation were distinctly reduced or not

308

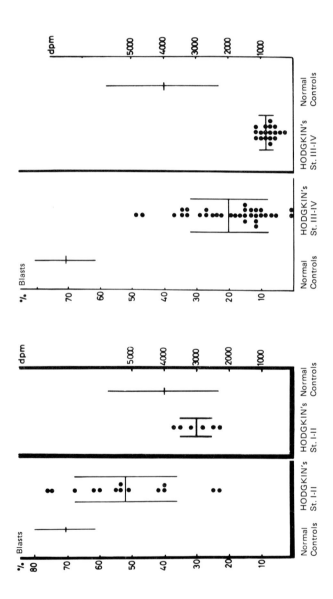

Fig. 1. Lymphocyte transformation [% blasts] and [^{14}C]-thymidine incorporation [dpm] in the 3-day PHA culture of lymphocytes of patients with lymphogranulomatosis, Stage I - II [left side of the figure] and Stage III - IV [right side of the figure].

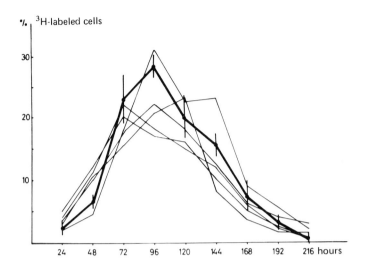

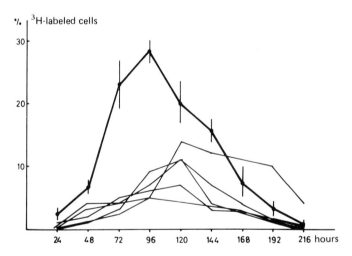

Fig.2. ^{3}H labelling index as a function of the incubation time of lymphocyte cultures from patients with lympho-granulomatosis, Stage I - II [upper part of the figure] and Stage III - IV [lower part of the figure]. The heavy line represents the average values from the control experiments.

detectable [Fig.1 and 2]. The relatively frequent appearance of macrophages was striking. The number of them was inversely proportional to the number of blast cells.

The ^{3}H index for cultivated lymphocytes from lymphogranulomatosis patients in Stage I - II was almost comparable with that
for the controls [Fig. 2]. In one Stage I case, the number of ^{3}H-
marked cells rose continuously from the 24th through the 96th
hour of incubation. The ^{3}H index was 32% in the 96th hour. The
lymphocytes from a patient in Stage II reached a peak of ^{3}H
labelling [23%] in the 120th hour of incubation. The number of
^{3}H-marked cells in the lymphocyte cultures from patients in the
advanced stages [III - IV] was significantly lower than in the
control during the entire observation time of more than 216 h
[Fig. 2].

The proliferation kinetics of the PHA-stimulated lymphocytes of
patients with lymphogranulomatoses were examined, yielding the
following data:

A. Lymphogranulomatoses, Stage I-II
    a] DNA-synthesis phase: 13.3 h
    b] Minimum length of the G2 phase: 2 h
    c] Actual generation time: 31.5 h

B. Lymphogranulomatoses, Stage III-IV
    a] DNA-synthesis: 13.47 h
    b] Minimum length of the G2 phase: 2 h
    c] Actual generation time: 39 h.

Lymphocytes from 10 patients with Morbus HODGKIN [3 in Stage
I or II and 7 in Stage III or IV] were separated out on a RABINO-
WITZ column and incubated for 264 h "in vivo" in a diffusion
chamber. Every 48 h, one chamber was removed for marking
with [methyl-^{3}H] thymidine and subsequent preparation of
smears. In contrast to the lymphocytes from patients with chronic lymphatic leukemia, with these HODGKIN's cells there was

no significant increase in the number of blasts after 120 or 146 h
[compare Fig. 8]. There was an increase in the number of blast-
like cells after 120 h incubation in just one case. The autoradiographic data correlated with the light microscopic observations;
the ^{3}H index corresponded in every case to the lymphocyte transformation rate [Fig. 3]. We did not observe an increase in the
incorporation of [3H] thymidine in advanced stages of the disease
[Fig. 3].

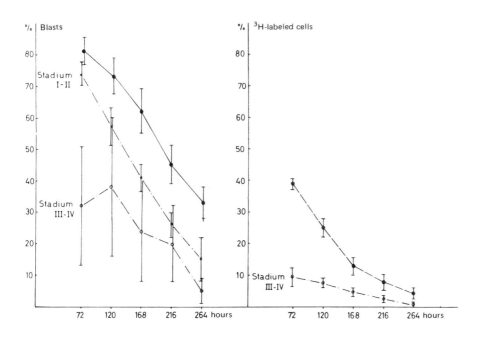

Fig. 3. Blast transformation and [3H] thymidine incorporation
in the diffusion chamber of lymphocytes from patients
with lymphogranulomatosis. The values are compared
to those from a normal control subject [solid line].

Stimulation of normal lymphocytes with PHA and specific antigens
in the presence of the plasma from lymphogranulomatosis
patients:

A. Controls:

If lymphocytes from healthy donors are incubated in the
presence of PHA with normal homologous plasma, there is
after 72 h a regular formation of blasts, or an incorporation
of [^{3}H] thymidine which corresponds to the standard experiment [cultivation of normal cells with autologous plasma]
[Fig. 4 and 5].

B. When normal lymphocytes were cultivated with HODGKIN's
disease plasma, an inhibition of the transformation was
observed after 72 h incubation [Fig. 4]. This inhibition was
dependent on the stage of the disease [Fig. 4]. Plasmas from
patients in advanced stages of the disease inhibited most
severely [Fig. 4].

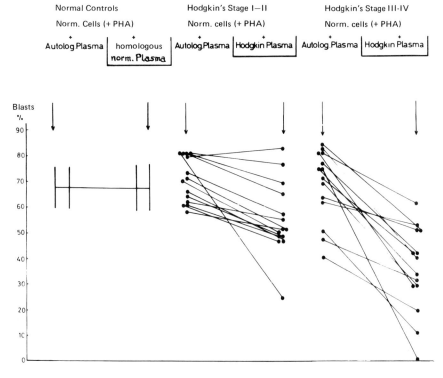

Fig. 4. The effect of an inhibitory factor in the plasma of lymphogranulomatosis patients on the PHA transformation of
normal lymphocytes.

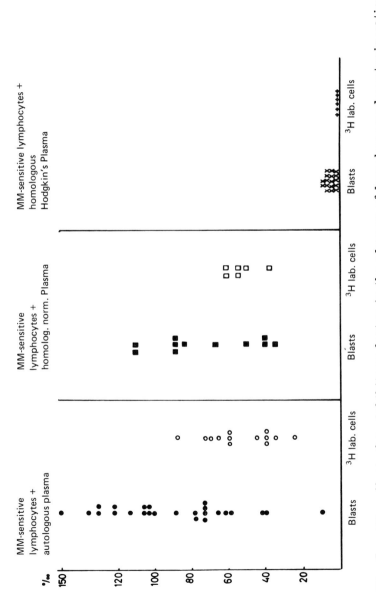

Fig. 5.   The effect of an inhibitory factor in the plasma of lymphogranulomatosis patients on the transformation of tuberculin-sensitive lymphocytes of healthy subjects [MM = MENDEL-MANTOUX]

In order to exclude an unspecific phytohemagglutinin reaction with the α_2M globulin of the HODGKIN's disease plasma [25], we also tested the effect of the plasma inhibition factor with the specific antigen model. Lymphocytes from MANTOUX-positive healthy subjects were incubated in the presence of tuberculin [PPD] for 120 h. This produced blast formation or [^{3}H] thymidine incorporation by the stimulated lymphocytes, when they were cultivated with autologous plasma, both at rates corresponding to the intensity of the skin reaction [Fig. 5]. The transformation was not affected by cultivation of the tuberculin-positive lymphocytes with homologous normal plasma [Fig. 5]. However, in 17 cases examined [Stages III-IV], there was little or no transformation when the normal MANTOUX-positive lymphocytes were cultivated with HODGKIN's disease plasma in the presence of PPD [Fig. 5]. Furthermore, it was striking that cytolysis was observed in more than half the cases.

2. Chronic lymphatic leukemias

There are distinct differences, with respect to transformation and [^{3}H] thymidine incorporation, between the lymphocytes from this group of patients and those from the controls. The number of blasts from two patients - one with high and one with low lymphocyte count - was 59% [Fig. 6]. The blast transformations from 14 patients were between 50 and 25%; from the others there were less than 20%. No significant differences were found between patients with high and low lymphocyte counts in the peripheral blood [Fig. 6].

^{3}H index: The ^{3}H index remained below the normal range over the entire observation period [216 h] [Fig. 7]. It was interesting that the highest ^{3}H indices [7.9 to 15.6%] were found for 4 patients with relatively low lymphocyte counts [between 11 200 and

30 000] [Fig. 7]. In most of the cases with low lymphocyte counts, the tritium labelling curve had two peaks, with a first maximum in the 72nd hour and a second in the 144th hour of incubation. In four cases of chronic lymphatic leukemia with more than 100 000 leucocytes in the peripheral blood, the number of labeled cells reached a maximum [4.5%] only after 120 h of incubation. Mitoses were seldom observed in the light microscope; the maximum also occured at 120 h.

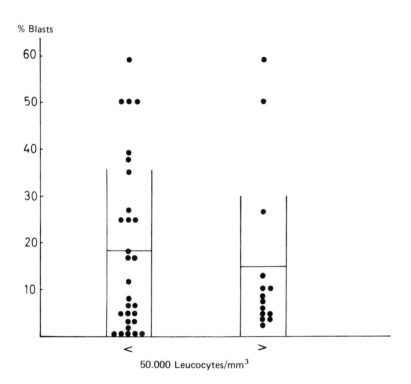

Fig. 6.   Relation of lymphocyte transformation and lymphocyte count in peripheral blood of patients with chronic lymphatic leukemia. The percentage of blasts in the 3-day culture is indicated.

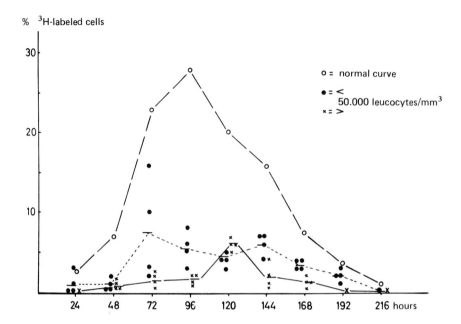

% ^{3}H-labeled cells

o = normal curve

● = < 50.000 leucocytes/mm^3

x = >

Fig.7. ^{3}H index as a function of the incubation time in the PHA
culture and the lymphocyte count in the peripheral blood
of patients with chronic lymphatic leukemia.

The proliferation rate studies on PHA-stimulated lymphocytes
from patients with chronic lymphatic leukemia yielded the following average values:

a] DNA-synthesis phase: 13.32 h

b] Minimum length of the G2 phase: 2 h

c] Actual generation time: 36 h.

The PHA-stimulated transformation in the diffusion chamber of
blood lymphocytes from patients with chronic lymphatic leukemia
was significantly reduced. Not only the number of transformed
cells, but also the rate of stimulation differed from those in
healthy controls: The number of blastocytes among the leukemic
lymphocytes only began to increase after 168 h [Fig. 8]. The ^{3}H

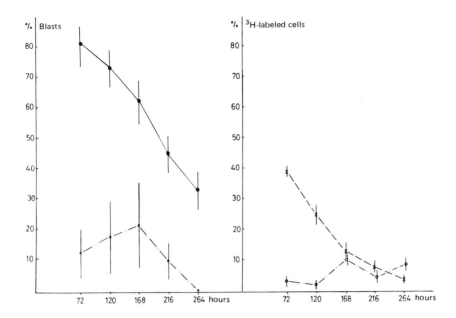

<u>Fig.8.</u>   Lymphocyte transformation [% blasts] and ^{3}H index
[^{3}H-labeled cells] in PHA-stimulated lymphocytes in
the diffusion chamber. The lymphocytes were taken
from patients with chronic lymphatic leukemia [broken
lines] or normal subjects [solid line].

incorporation in the cells cultivated in vivo [^{3}H index] indicated
a delay in DNA synthesis [Fig. 8]. The lymphocyte transformation remained low for more than 264 h in only one case with a
very high lymphocyte count [300 000 /mm^3] in the peripheral
blood. In the other cases, the number of blasts formed [or the
^{14}C thymidine incorporated] was in the normal proportion to the
leukocyte number.

3.   Lymphocyte transformation in <u>cases of stomach ulcers and</u>
<u>stomach carcinomas:</u>
In 25 cases of stomach or duodenal ulcer, the [^{14}C] thymidine
incorporation of the cultivated leukocytes was in the normal

range [Fig. 9]. The [^{14}C]thymidine incorporation was very low [820 dpm] in only one case [stomach ulcer with complicating fungal infection]. In contrast to this group, the [^{14}C]thymidine incorporation of lymphocytes from all examined patients with stomach carcinoma was significantly reduced [p < 0.0005], with the exception of 5 patients with microcarcinomas of the stomach. The diagnoses were histologically confirmed from operation

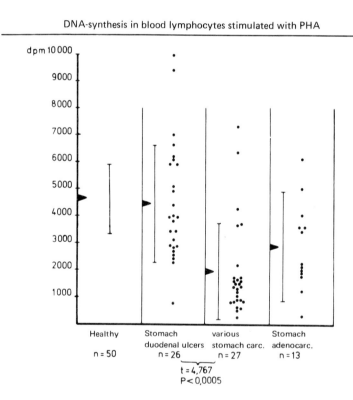

Fig. 9. [^{14}C]thymidine incorporation after 3-day incubation by blood lymphocytes of normal controls, patients with stomach-duodenal ulcers and patients with stomach carcinomas or adenocarcinomas.

biopsies. The lymphocytes of 6 patients with adenocarcinomas of
the stomach underwent normal transformation [Fig. 9]. On the
average, however, the [^{14}C] thymidine incorporation of the cultivated lymphocytes was moderately reduced compared to the controls, although not as much as in the stomach carcinoma group
[Fig. 9].

4. Isolation of an inhibiting factor in the plasma of patients with
malignant tumors:

Earlier investigations in our laboratory indicated that the plasma
of carcinoma patients strongly influences not only the PHA transformation of normal lymphocytes, but also the blast formation or
[^{3}H] thymidine incorporation of PPD-stimulated lymphocytes of
tuberculin-positive subjects [11]. After chromatographic separation of the serum from patients, the inhibitory factor was found
in fraction IV. The fractions I, II and III were incapable of inhibiting the blast transformation [Fig. 10 and 11]. The inhibitory
factor was found in all cases of lymphogranulomatosis, metastasizing tumors, acute leukemia, and in the two examined cases
of gravidity. It was not detectable, either in the whole plasma or
in its fractions, in healthy subjects, chronic lymphatic leukemia,
chronic myeloic leukemia or in four cases of stomach adenocarcinoma which had had a normal [^{14}C]thymidine incorporation in
the PHA culture [compare Fig. 9].

Discussion

Lymphogranulomatosis is the prototype of a disease with a
defective cellular immune system. The immunological compe-
tence of patients with Morbus HODGKIN has been intensively
investigated in the last 20 years. It has been confirmed by numerous observations that in these patients there is a reduced

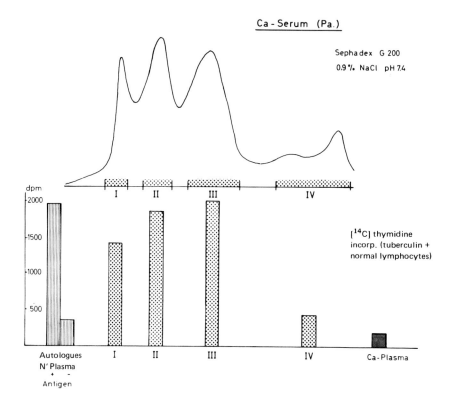

Fig. 10. Chromatography of the serum of a patient with stomach
carcinoma on Sephadex G-200 [0.1 M Tris, pH 7.4]. The
effect of the fractions and the whole plasma on the
transformation[[^{14}C] thymidine incorporation] of tuberculin-sensitive lymphocytes. The inhibitory factor is
found in Fraction IV.

cellular immune reaction [20,26-31]. Among other things, a delay in the rejection of skin transplants [32,33] and a disturbed
lymphocyte function [34-39] were observed. In contrast to the
lymphoproliferative diseases, there is no impairment of the
humoral immune reactions, so that the primary and secondary
immune response in these patients seems to be intact [27,40].

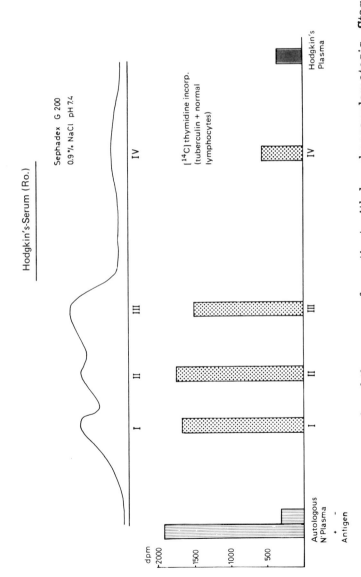

Fig. II. Chromatography of the serum of a patient with lymphogranulomatosis, Stage IV, on Sephadex G-200 [0.1 M Tris, pH 7.4]. Effect of the fractions and the whole plasma on the transformation of tuberculin-sensitized lymphocytes. The inhibitory factor is found in Fraction IV.

While some research groups [29,30,32] found an anergic state in 45 or 100% of their patients, others [40,41] reported that the delayed epicutaneous reactions were negative in only 16% or 26.6% of their untreated lymphogranulomatosis patients. It is possibly that this discrepancy is due to differences in the basis for selection of appropriate subjects. The cellular immune reaction is seldom affected in the early stages of the disease; the defects only appear in the later stages [III - IV].

Lymphocyte transformation and [^{3}H or ^{14}C] thymidine incorporation were, as a rule, reduced with our patients, and the degree depended on the stage of the disease. In all Stage III and IV patients the reaction was greatly diminished. HERSH and OPPENHEIM [34] also reported a reaction of the peripheral lymphocytes of HODGKIN's Disease patients which depended on the progress of the disease and was correlated with its stages. The observations described in the literature range from normal to moderately reduced transformation ability of the blood lymphocytes [35, 41-44], and sometimes even include premature death of the culture [32,34,39]. In the majority of cases of Morbus HODGKIN, however, a slight amount of blast formation in PHA-stimulated blood lymphocytes is reported.

In our long-term cultures in vitro, we found, in agreement with other authors [41], a maximum of DNA synthesis at 120 h after the beginning of the incubation, which is later than observed with normal controls. This applied only to Stage III or IV. In these experiments we did not observe a two-peaked course of DNA duplication activity as reported by HAVEMANN and SCHMIDT [41] and suggested by them to be due to an additional early reaction of the lymphocytes which depended on the lymphocyte count in the peripheral blood. Studies of the prolifer-

ation kinetics of stimulated lymphocytes of lymphogranulomatosis
patients revealed that the length of the DNA-synthesis phase and
the G2 phase were the same as those of healthy subjects or patients with chronic lymphatic leukemia. In general there was a
constant DNA-synthesis time and G2 phase in all the cultures
examined, an observation which agrees with the results from
numerous autoradiographic studies on healthy and tumor cells.
It appears that the time period from the beginning of the DNA
synthesis phase to the end of mitosis is subject to relatively
little variation. Differences in the generation time are for the
most part due to variations in the G1 phase [42-44].

The actual generation time of PHA-stimulated lymphocytes from
patients with lymphogranulomatosis was not significantly longer
than that of cells from healthy controls. Since the generation
time was extended in only one case [Stage IV], it does not seem
justifiable, in light of the present results, to assume that the
defective cellular immune reaction usually observed in advanced
cases of lymphogranulomatosis is generally due to an increase
in the generation time of the immunologically competent cells.
It seems more likely that in HODGKIN's disease, a reduction
in the number of immunologically competent cells is responsible
for the defect. Indeed, the observation that the proliferation
kinetics of lymphocytes from patients with chronic lymphatic
leukemia and lymphogranulomatosis are about the same as the
controls suggests that the defects in the immune reaction observed in both diseases are not due to the presence of lymphocytes with abnormal proliferation kinetics, but rather to the
reduction in the number of cells which have normal proliferation reactions. In chronic lymphatic leukemia, the decisive
factor seems to be the crowding out of healthy, normally pro-

liferating cells by leukemic cell clones, whereas in lympho-granulomatosis, it may be that some of the cells are so changed that they lose their immunological reactivity. Both our electron microscopic observations and the experimental results of other research groups suggest a cell defect [45]. FAZIO and BACHI [46] achieved an increased transformation of lymphocytes, corresponding to the normal controls, by adding RNA extracted from the leucocytes of normal persons to inactive HODGKIN cultures [24 h after the beginning of the incubation]. Thus it is possible that the decreased PHA reaction is the result of a lack of or defect in a particular RNA, which can still exercise its function after 24 h and bring the pathological lymphocytes into a normal biological cell cycle. Another indication that a cell defect is involved are the cytoplasmic extensions of the lymphocytes, which are a typical symptom of dying cells.

Our results with the lymphocyte transformation in patients with chronic lymphatic leukemia agree well with the results of other research groups, where in some cases transformation rates of 20% after 3 to 4 days' incubation were reported [47-54]. We found no relationship between the transformation rate and the peripheral leucocyte count or the immunoglobulin concentration in the serum [39], but other authors have described a correlation between peripheral lymphocyte count and blast formation in the PHA culture [50,54,55]. We did find one reaction which was a function of the lymphocyte count, but only in our long-term cultures which were done by the diffusion chamber method. However, there was no significant difference in the blast transformation in cultures from treated and untreated patients. Other investigators have also found no effect of the glucocorticosteroid or cytostatic therapies on the blast formation in culture [53,56].

An increase in the lymphocyte transformation was only achieved by irradiation of the spleen with a total of 300 - 600 r, but the effect was transitory and fell off again after 2 - 4 weeks [57].

Patients with chronic lymphatic leukemia differ from healthy controls not only in the number of blast-like transformed cells and the [^{14}C or ^{3}H] thymidine incorporation of the stimulated lymphocytes, but also in the fine structure of the cells. It can be seen with an electron microscope that the PHA cells among the leukemic lymphocytes after 3 days' culture are larger than the unstimulated lymphocytes, have a chromatin-rich nucleus with 1 or 2 nucleoli, and have more mitochondria and other cell organelles in the cytoplasm [45]. These small transformed cells are also characterized by a very low RNA and polyribosome concentration, and either do not transform into blastoid forms, or do so seldom. In our material we found no blasts with typical fine structure. It was noticeable that the leukemic stimulated lymphocytes lacked any sign of phagocytotic activity such as lipid inclusions or vacuoles [45]. Macrophages were also lacking in our cultures, whether examined by light or electron microscopy. In the case of chronic lymphatic leukemia, the transformation seemed to be blocked in the initial stages. However, in the long-term cultures in vitro and in the diffusion chamber, there was a late transformation and an increased DNA synthesis in the leukemic cells, as was also found by HAVEMANN and RUBIN [58]. Various possible causes of the reduced transformability have been discussed. ASTALDI et al. [59] originally reported a plasma factor in the serum of chronic lymphatic leukemia patients which inhibited the transformation of normal lymphocytes. However, further experiments by the same research group failed to confirm these results [60]. KASAKURA

and LOWENSTEIN [51] even claimed that the plasma of patients
with chronic lymphatic leukemia is capable of activating normal
lymphocytes to blastogenesis and DNA synthesis. The reduced
PHA-stimulated transformability in vitro of blood lymphocytes
from patients with chronic lymphatic leukemia is in all probability due to a cell defect.

In agreement with other authors [62], we found a reduction in
blast transformation and [^{14}C]thymidine incorporation in PHA-
stimulated lymphocytes from untreated patients with malignant,
non-lymphoreticular diseases [11]. Our examination of patients
with stomach carcinomas revealed a significantly reduced [^{14}C]
thymidine incorporation of the cultivated blood lymphocytes.
The lymphocyte reaction to PHA was most strongly curtailed in
cases of metastasizing tumors [12]. This leads to the suspicion
that tumor growth and metastases are favored by the weakened
immune defense. Although the results of lymphocyte transformation in vitro imply a relationship between impaired cellular
immune reaction and tumor growth, the question of the primary
mutual influences cannot be answered by experiments on organisms which are already diseased. Experiments on NMRI mice
with EHRLICH ascites and solid tumors of the EHRLICH ascites
type indicated that the course of the immune reaction is not
changed by tumor development, but its extent is limited [11].

The plasma of patients with lymphogranulomatosis or malignant,
non-lymphoreticular diseases inhibited both PHA-induced and
specific-antigen-stimulated transformation of normal lymphocytes in vitro [62-64]. This inhibition cannot be due to an unspecific phytohemagglutinin reaction with the α_2M globulin of
the HODGKIN or carcinoma plasma, since the inhibitory effect
of the plasma from patients with lymphogranulomatosis or tu-

mors was also observed with tuberculin-stimulated lymphocyte cultures [lymphocytes from healthy subjects who were oversensitive to the MENDEL-MANTOUX test]. The cause of the reduced reaction of lymphocytes to PHA in patients with Morbus HODGKIN and tumors is therefore not a cell defect alone, but also a plasmatic factor. After chromatographic separation of the serum of these patients on Sephadex G-200, we determined that only one fraction [peak IV] can inhibit transformation. From the chromatographic analysis it can be assumed that the inhibitory factor has a low molecular weight, but we know nothing more about it at present. It could be a peptide or a nucleoprotein.

Observation of the course of the disease in patients with various malignant tumors indicated that the lymphocyte transformation test has a certain predictive value [66]. According to CORDER et al. [65], there is no correlation between the intensity of the blast transformation in the presence of PHA in vitro and the length of survival of HODGKIN's Disease patients. Although the test is thus incapable of giving information about the prognosis, it is in general a valuable index of the immunological status of these patients.

Summary

The ability of blood lymphocytes to transform into blast-like cells in the presence of phytohemagglutinin serves as a model for the cellular immune reaction. The ability is reduced in the peripheral-blood lymphocytes of patients with lymphogranulomatosis, chronic lymphatic leukemia or carcinoma. In HODGKIN's Disease, the degree of the transformation depends on the stage of the disease. The cause of the decreased lymphocyte reaction to phytohemagglutinin in patients with Morbus HODGKIN and tumors is not only a cellular defect of the lymphocytes, but is also the presence of a plasmatic inhibitory factor.

References

1. MORTON,D.L.[1971],J.Reticuloendothelial Soc.10,137

2. HELLSTRÖM,I.,HELLSTRÖM,K.E.,SJÖGREN,H.O. & WARNER,G.A. [1971], Int.J.Cancer 7,1

3. KLEIN,G.[1971],Israel J.Med.Sci. 7, 111

4. DIEHL,V.,JEREB,B.,STJERNSWÄRD,J.,O'TOLLE,C. & ÅHSTRÖM,L. [1971],Int.J.Cancer 7, 277

5. SEGALL,A.,WILER,O.,GENIM,J.,LACOUR,J. & LACOUR,F.[1972], Int.J.Cancer 4, 417

6. YOUNG,R.C.,CORDER,M.P.,HAYNES,H.A.& DE VITA, V.T. [1972], Amer.J.Med. 52,63

7. BAKKEREN,J.A.J.,DE VAAD,G.A.M. & SCHRETLEN, E.D.A.N. [1972], Scand.J.Haematol. 9, 36

8. FAIRLEY,G.H.[1969], Brit.Med.J. 2, 467

9. HELLSTRÖM,I.,HELLSTRÖM,K.E.,PIERCE,G.E. & YANG,J.P.S.[1968], Nature [London] 220, 1352

10. SMITH,R.T.[1968], N.Engl.J.Med.278, 1207,1268,1326

11. SCHEURLEN,P.G. & PAPPAS,A.[1971],Verh.Deut.Ges. Inn.Med. 77, 749

12. SCHEURLEN,P.G. [1971], Med.Welt 22 [N.F.] 1257

13. BURNET,F.M. [1967], Lancet I, 1171

14. GOOD,R.A.[1970], Hosp.Pract. 5, 9

15. KLEIN,G.[1966], Ann.Rev.Microbiol. 20, 223

16. KLEIN,G.[1968], Cancer Res. 28, 625

17. WANTED,H.J.,ZIPP,P.A. & KOUNTZ,S.L.[1969],Surg. Forum 20, 120

18. GOOD,P.A.[1967], Experimental and clinical experiences with chemical suppression of immunity, in Immunopathology, 5th Internat.Symposium, p.366 and 416 [eds.Miescher,P.A. & Grabar,P.] Grune & Stratton, New York

19. PENN,I.[1970], Malignant tumors in organ transplant recipients, in Recent Results in Cancer Research, Springer-Verlag, Berlin - Heidelberg - New York

20. SCHEURLEN,P.G.[1971], Vortrag, Immunologische Probleme bei der Lymphogranulomatose, Deut.Krebskongreß, Hannover

21. LEWIN,A.G.,McDONOUGH,E.F.jr.,MILLER,D.G. & SOUTHEN,Ch.M. [1964], Ann.N.Y.Acad.Sci. 120,400

22. LEWIN,A.G.,GUSTODIO,D.B.,MANDEL,E.E. & SOUTHAM,G.M. [1964], Ann.N.Y.Acad.Sci. 120, 410

23. PAPPAS,A. & SCHEURLEN,P.G.[1972],Lymphocyte Transformation in Malignant Diseases. Communication I: Methodologic Problems, This issue

24. PERRY,S.[1967], Ann.Internal Med. 67, 424

25. HAVEMANN,K.,DOSCH,H.N. & BÜRGER,S.[1970],Z. Gesamte Exp.Med. 153, 297 and 308

26. SCHIER,W.W.[1954], N.Engl.J.Med. 250, 353

27. CHASE,M.W. [1966], Cancer Res. 26, 1097

28. AISENBERG,A.C.[1962], J.Clin.Invest. 41,1964

29. SCHIER,W.W.,ROTH,A.,OSTROFF,G. & SCHRIFT,M. [1965], Amer.J.Med. 20, 94

30. LAMB,D.,PILNEY,F.,KELLY,W.D. & GOOD,R.A.[1962], J.Immunol. 89, 555

31. SOKAL,J.E. & PRIMIKIRIOS,N.[1961], Cancer 14, 597

32. KELLY,W.D.,LAMB,D.L.,VARCO,R.L. & GOOD,R.A. [1960],Ann.N.Y.Acad.Sci. 87, 187

33. KELLY,W.D., GOOD,R.A. & VARCO,R.L.[1958],Surg. Gynec.Obstet.107,565

34. HERSH,E.M. & OPPENHEIM,J.J.[1965], N.Engl.J.Med. 273, 1006

35. AISENBERG,A.C.[1965], J.Clin.Invest. 44, 555

36. PAPAC,R.J. [1970], Cancer 26, 279

37. JACKSON,S.M.,GARRETT,J.V. & GRAIG,A.W.[1970], Cancer 25, 843

38. HAN, T. & SOKAL, J.E.[1970], Amer.J.Med. 48,728

39. SCHEURLEN, P.G., PAPPAS, A. & LUDWIG, T.[1968], Klin. Wochenschr. 46, 483

40. BROWN, R.S., HAYNES, H.A., FOLEX, H.T., GODWIN, H.A., BERARD, C.W. & CARBONE, P.P.[1967], Ann. Intern. Med. 67, 291

41. HAVEMANN, K. & SCHMIDT, M.[1968], Klin. Wochenschr. 46, 31

42. MENDELSON, M.L., DOHAN, F.C. & MOORE, H.A.[1960], J.Nat. Cancer Inst. 28, 477

43. CATTANEO, S.M., QUASTLER, H. & SHERMAN, F.C.[1961], Nature [London] 190, 923

44. PILGRIM, Ch. & MAURER, W. [1962], Naturwissenschaften 49, 544

45. PAPPAS, A., ORFANOS, C. & SCHEURLEN, P.G.[1969], Z. Gesamte Exp. Med. 149, 294

46. FAZIO, M. & BACHI, G.[1967], Nature [London] 215, 629

47. SCHREK, R. & RABINOWITZ, Y.[1963], Proc. Soc. Exp. Med. Biol. 113, 191

48. SCHREK, R., FRIEDMAN, I.A. & LEITHOLD, S.L.[1958], J.Nat. Cancer Inst. 20, 1037

49. ASTALDI, G.[1964], Med. Klin. 59, 368

50. BERNARD, C., GERALDES, A. & BOIRON, M.[1964], Nouv. Rev. Franç. d'Hematol. 4, 69

51. QUAGLINO, D. & COWLING, D.C. [1964], Brit. J. Haematol. 10, 358

52. ROBBINS, J.H.[1964a], Experientia 20, 164

53. ASTALDI, G., COSTA, G. & AIRO, R.[1965], Lancet II, 1394

54. GROPP, A. & KLEE, F.[1969], Verh. Deut. Ges. Pathol. 53, 503

55. RUBIN, A.D., HAVEMANN, K. & DAMESHEK, W.[1969], Blood, 33, 313

56. OPPENHEIM, J.J., WHANG, J. & FREI, E.[1965], Blood 26, 121

57. ASTALDI, G., AIRO, R., COSTA, G. & DUARTE, N.[1965b], Lancet II, 905

58. HAVEMANN,K. & RUBIN,A.D.[1968],Proc.Soc.Exp.Biol. Med. 127,668

59. ASTALDI,G.,COSTA,G. & AIRO,R.[1965c],Lancet I,1394

60. ASTALDI,G. & AIRO,R.[1967],Phytohaemagglutinin and human lymphocytes in short-term cell culture, in The Lymphocyte in Immunology and Haemopoiesis [ed.Yoffey, J.M.] Edward Arnold, London

61. KASAKURA,A. & LOWENSTEIN,L.[1967],Blood 29,691

62. SILK,M.[1967], Cancer 20, 2088

63. TRUBOWITZ,S.,MASEK,B. & DEL ROSARIO,A.[1966], Cancer 19,2019

64. SCHEURLEN,P.G.,PAPPAS,A. & LUDWIG,T.[1968], Klin.Wochenschr. 46, 483

65. CORDER,M.P.,YOUNG,R.C.,BROWN,R.S. & DE VITA, V.T. [1972],Blood 39, 595

66. CHEEMA,A.R. & HERSH,E.M.[1971],Cancer 28, 851

6.2 Immunosuppressive Therapy with Anti-lymphocytic Globulin and Tumor Formation

W. Brendel and J. Ring

BURNET's hypothesis, dating back to 1959 [1], that formation
and growth of tumors depend on the immunological reactivity of
the organism, was basically theoretical. In the meantime this
theory, which implicates that neoplasms only arise if they are
able to evade the immunological system, has been proved by
experimental and clinical research. This means that tumor cells
have different antigenic patterns from normal host cells. Tumor
cells which are transplanted into a syngeneic organism are regarded as an allograft and trigger an immune response leading
to their rejection. The spontaneous and environment induced
cancerogenic mutations, which take place continuously, do not
evoque a clinical tumor formation for the only reason that a
healthy organism will kill those "degenerated" cells immediately.
As a matter of fact humoral and cellular immune reactions could
be demonstrated in numerous animal experiments after transplantation of a chemically or virus induced tumor into a genetically identical host, as well as in some human tumorous diseases,
e.g. BURKITT's lymphoma, melanoma, neuroblastoma, sarcoma
and adenocarcinoma [2,3,4].

For this consideration the cause of the tumor specific antigen
deviation does not matter: A special virus may have infected the
cell, an oncogenic virus may have changed the genoma of the
tumor cells, finally chemical, physical or "spontaneous" factors
may have initiated the tumor specific change of a cell's antigenic
pattern [i.e. the protein stucture].

The important fact is the real difference in antigenicity between
tumor and normal cells. In Table 1 the hitherto described ways of
such "tumor-specific" antigen variables are enlisted: Except the
saprophytic virus infections, always changes in the genoma of the
cell are the causative factors, whether it is a true, new information transfer by RNA or DNA viruses, or the derepression of an
existing but blocked genoma or the appearance of HL-A-differences.
Some examples may demonstrate the hypothesis: Cell of BUR-
KITT's lymphoma, of some carcinomas of the pharynx as well
as of infectious mononucleosis, show an antigenicity which is
evoqued by viruses of the BARR-EBSTEIN resp. the HERPES
group. Recently the incorporation of nuclear acids of the BARR-
EBSTEIN virus into the genoma of the human host cell could be demonstrated [5]. A possible viral etiology of melanoma is discussed,
too [6]; however, there have been found different antigenic determinants in melanoma cells at the same time. The demonstration
of tumor specific fetal proteins [superficial antigens], which was
possible in human adenocarcinoma and hepatoma, might be of
diagnostic importance. α- and γ-fetoproteins are not tumor
specific; they are also observed in diseases with high rate of
cell decay [7].

Teratoid tumors [chorio-epithelioma resp. - carcinoma] are
true allogeneic transplants, i.e. the antigenic difference results
out of genetic difference in the HL-A-pattern between teratoid
and host cell.

According to experimental and clinical findings, the genesis of
such "tumor-specific" antigens obeys to the following principles
[Table 1].

1] In histologically different tissues of different individuals of the
same species the same virus induces the same antigens, which
do not depend on individual nor cell type. The occuring antibodies
are cross-reacting with the inducing virus.

Table 1 : Possible " tumor-specific" antigens

cause	mechanism	antigen	example
virus	viral genoma	virus, not tumor-specific	BURKITT's lymphoma
		neoantigen, group-specific	sarcoma [mouse]
viral, chemical or physical influences	true change in the genoma of a cell	neoantigen, individual and group-specific	various tumors [mouse, rat, human]
	activation resp.	carcino-embryonic antigen	colonic carcinoma [human]
	derepression of a	α-fetoprotein	hepatoma [human]
	blocked genoma	γ-fetoprotein	various tumors [human]
		TL-antigen	leukemia [mouse]
conception	genetic difference from maternal cell	HL-A-antigen	chorio-epithelioma [human]
spontaneous mutations	change of a genoma	?	?

2] Another kind of individual independent antigenicity can be demonstrated in some tumors together with the appearance of carcino-embryonic or fetal proteins. This derepression of genetic information may be produced by chemical, physical or viral influences. The occuring antibodies are not tumor-specific; crossreactions with pathologically changed, but not neoplastic tissue are possible.

3] True tumor-specific neoantigens may be induced by physical and chemical influences. Cell- and tumor-specific - i.e. crossrecating with other tumors - antibodies are observed.

4] The teratoid tumors [chorio-.epithelioma resp.-carcinoma] show HL-A antigens which differ from the HL-A pattern of the organism. The occuring antibodies are classical transplantation antibodies.

These introductory and incomplete remarks on the specific antigenicity of tumor tissue may only explain that the immunological control of tumor growth is scientifically proved and not only of theoretical but of clinical diagnostic or even therapeutical importance; however, it must be mentioned that there are still a lot of human tumors without proved antigenic specifity; there even may exist some neoplasms, which show the contrary, i.e. a reduced number of transplantation antigens [and which perhaps therefore evade the control mechanism of the host].

The growth of all tumors, which show an antigenicity different from that of the host organism, is only possible under certain well defined conditions:

I. The antigenicity of the tumor cell must be too weak to trigger an immunological defence reaction. Weak transplantation antigens may produce - as in the transplantation of genetically similar tissue - a "sneak-through-phenomenon", i.e. the immune reaction does not exceed the level, which could lead to a tumor threatening production of cytotoxic antibodies.

II. The antigenicity and the growth of the tumor cells is so strong, that the immune defence system of the host is over challenged and not able to prevent tumor growth despite of stimulation.

III. Despite of an existing antigenic difference of the tumor cell there is no immune reaction, because the host organism is immunologically tolerant against the tumor antigen - or the tumor inducing virus.

IV. The immune system of the host is stimulated by the tumor antigen, but produces not only cytotoxic, but also protective antibodies resp. factors [8-10]. Such enhancement phenomena are well known in tumor immunology.

V. The immune defence system of the host is pathologically weakened, e.g. in thymus aplasia, agammaglobulinemia or after severe infections.

VI. The immune system of the host is blocked by therapeutical procedures [X-rays, antibiotics, immunosuppressives].

All these 6 possibilities are experimentally and clinically proved. In the following only point VI, the influence of immunosuppression with particular emphasis on ALG shall be discussed. The other above mentioned factors must never be neglected.

If there is an immunological control of tumor formation and growth at all, any weakening of the immune system should lead to an accumulation of tumor production and an increase of tumor growth. The experimental model of immunological weakness is the condition after pre- or neonatal thymectomy, which results in a reduction of the number of T-lymphocytes and a generalized lymphocytic hypoplasia. In this condition an increased rate of

spontaneous tumor formation [11-14] as well as a facilitated growth
of chemically or virus induced tumors has been observed [1,11,
15 - 21]. Contrary observations may be caused by species differences or by the too late performance of neonatal thymectomy
[22]. Azathioprine, too, the most frequently used immunosuppressive drug, induces an increase in spontaneous tumor rate
[16,23]. The spontaneous formation of an adenocarcinoma, after
prolongued administration of Azathioprine and Prednisolone has
been described in dogs [24]. It is astonishing that about the tumor
facilitating effect of Azathioprine and steroids so little experimental work has been done, however still more than about the
effect of X-rays in the doses in which they are used in immunosuppressive treatment. HARAN-GHERA could show that after
treatment with an oncogenic extract out of radiated bone marrow,
tumors in the transplanted thymus of sublethally radiated mice
took root easier than in unradiated animals [25].

In comparison to that, extensive experimental studies have been
performed with the most powerful immunosuppressive, Antilymphocytic Globulin. Several authors agree that during ALG
therapy tumors may be easier produced by oncogenic viruses,
and that these tumors are growing faster [11, 15,16,26,27]. The
same has been reported about chemical carcinogens [Methyl-
cholanthrene and ALS [28,29]].

NELSON's experiments illustrate the difficulties in judging the
tumor facilitating effect of ALS: The author found that the "spontaneous" occuring tumors during ALS-therapy over 12 months
were induced by a polioma virus, which was contained in a definite charge of rat-anti-mouse ALS [30]. By the way, all animals
- with or without tumors - developed humoral antibodies against
Polioma-virus. The application of ALS or ALG over periods of

weeks or months without simultaneous administration of an oncogenic - viral chemical or radiological - never induces tumor formation according to the results of numerous authors. ALS or ALG has therefore no true oncogenic effect [16,29,31]. This is confirmed by our own monotherapy studies with ALS [28], which we have performed during the last years on dogs and rats; for in no case we were able to observe a tumor formation.

Therefore, if the formation of neoplasms is observed in patients treated either conventionally with Azathioprine or steroids, or with ALG, one should carefully examine, whether carcinogenic factors are involved such as oncogenic viruses or proliferation interfering drugs as Azathioprine. A transfer of oncogenic viruses by ALG batches has not yet been observed in men. So it must be emphasized that ALS-therapy facilitated tumor formation and growth only, if this tumor has been produced by oncogenics; by ALG- or ALS-treatment per se no tumor formation can be induced - opposite to Azathioprine and other immunosuppressives. But even if a specific carcinogenic agent is present, ALG treatment does not necessarily increase the tumor risk. This can be concluded from studies of BALNER [32] in mice, who observed a lesser incidence of leukemia after irradiation if subsequently ALG was administered. This can be seen in Fig. 1: Curves 2 and 3 symbolyze the relative decrease in tumor production of ALG treated animals, compared to the controls, curve No. 1. These data may support the contention that immunosuppressive procedures per se not necessarily enhance a general attenuation of the immunological tumor defence.

According to experimental data, neoplasms of the lymphatic system are less likely to develop during ALG treatment compared to control conditions or to animals subjected to conventional im-

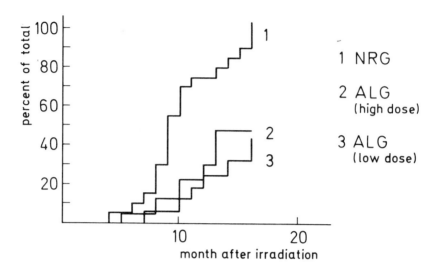

Fig.1. Effect of ALG-treatment on the incidence of "leukemia"
in ♂ RFM mice following single dose of 300 R.

munosuppression. However, it appears to be obvious, that much
more conclusive experiments have to be done in order to find out
the effect of immunosuppressive treatment on the formation and
growth of tumors.

The uncertainty concerning the influence of immunosuppression
on tumors will probably be increased by the findings of HELL-
STRÖM [8-10]. It is conceivable that certain immunosuppressive
methods affect the formation of tumor enhancing antibodies,
provided that these enhancing factors or antibodies described by
HELLSTRÖM can be identified as gamma globulins . It may be
visualized, that immunosuppression not only weakens the immunological tumor control, but enhances the immunological defence,
e.g. by destruction of tumor protecting antibodies, provided a
specific suppression of tumor antibodies can be excluded [Fig. 2].
In view of this argument, immunosuppressive therapy may be
considered as a method, capable to interfere with a possible

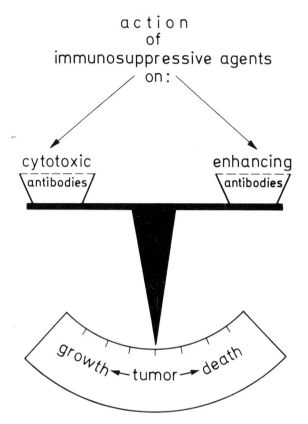

Fig. 2. Possible effects of immunosuppressive treatment on the balance between cytotoxic and blocking antibody formation and tumor growth.

equilibrium between tumor defence and tumor enhancement. Thus, it may be a matter of special circumstances, in which way the balance is disturbed by a particular drug. At the moment, we do not have any informations, how ALG or other immunosuppressive drugs may affect this delicate balance.

Comparable to the experimental findings in thymectomized animals are the well known accumulations in humans, whose immunological defence is reduced, as in various types of a- or hypogammaglobulinemia, morbus WALDENSTRÖM, plasmacytoma, WISKOTT-AL-

DRICH-syndrom etc. [33]. PENN and STARZL [34,35] were the first who reported 1968 and 1969 [36,37] an increased frequency of neoplasms among organ transplant recipients, who underwent immunosuppressive treatment. Since that time all such cases occurring in the USA are registered, and recently they have been published by PENN [34,35]: Among these tumors 44 are of epethelial and 32 of mesenchymal origin, which are enlisted in table 2. The most striking fact of this statistic is the low rate of the otherwise quite frequent tumors of lung, bronchia and mamma. [Are the oncogenic factors for such tumors reduced under the conditions of organ transplantation, or is it an unknown selection mechanism?].

Table 2:

Malignant tumors in organ homograft
recipients [world experience]   +], ++]

Types of tumors

I.	Epithelial tumors	44
	Skin tumors	11
	Carcinoma in situ of cervix	8
	Carcinoma of lip	8
	Lung tumors	4
	Hepatoma	2
	Miscellaneous carcinomas	11
II.	Mesenchymal tumors	32 x]
	Reticulum cell sarcoma	21
	Lymphoma	4
	KAPOSI's sarcoma	3
	Leiomyosarcoma	2
	Rhabdomyosarcoma	1
	Synovial sarcoma	1

x]Includes a patient with 2 tumors - a reticulum cell
   sarcoma of the brain and a KAPOSI's sarcoma of the
   skin.

+] according to PENN [34]
++] the percentage of these tumors compared to all organ
    transplant recipients cannot be described exactly,
    because there are not all cases registered by the
    World Organtransplant Registry

On the other hand, tumors of highly proliferating tissues are prevailing, which fact could suggest spontaneous mutations which are not averted during immunosuppressive therapy. At this time it is not possible to demonstrate, for which percentage of the world tumor statistic the tumors of table 2 stand, because the statistic of organ transplants is still incomplete. PENN and STARZL [35] observed among 352 recipients of kidney transplants of the University of Colorado, Medical Centre, and the Veteran's Administration Hospital, Denver, Colorado, 16 cases of tumors. With regards to 65 patients, who died of a variety of complications during the first 4 months, this number corresponds to a corrected tumor frequency of 5,6%, in comparison to a tumor rate of 0,058% among a control group of the same age. There exists another smaller statistic from the Peter Bent Brigham Hospital, Boston, with a [corrected] tumor rate of 3 - 3,5%.

A first objection towards the statistics of PENN is, that in the early years of organ transplantation cadaver kidneys have been used, originating from donors who died from tumors. Thus, malignant cells could have been transplanted and the growth of those cells might have been favoured by the immunosuppressive treatment [38,39], as seen in many animal experiments, too. Consequently, organs of tumor patients should be ruled out for transplantation as long as there is no way to separate the malignant cells from the grafted organ. In 2 cases a regression of the transplanted tumor could be achieved by early diagnosis and stop of immunosuppressive treatment [40-41] - a convincing example of the "immune surveillance" of tumor growth and the role of immunosuppression in men. The accumulation of epithelial surface tumors in the study [especially tumors of the skin] might be due to the fact that a relatively high number of people living in southern countries with a high intensity of sun exhibition were among the observed patients.

Regarding the special etiology, the problem remains unsolved, whether in the etiology of tumors oncogenic viruses play a decisive role, although we do not know yet, whether those viruses like the BARR-EPSTEIN virus or the Herpes Hominis II are really responsible for tumor formation.

STARZL as well as the Australian group have stated that according to their experiences the frequency of tumor formation was significantly reduced since Antilymphocytic Globulin was introduced into immunosuppressive therapy. STARZL believes that the reduction of tumor formation is due to the fact that ALG therapy permits a reduction of Prednisolone and Azathioprine. That could imply that the increase of tumor formation during immunosuppressive treatment is linked to the above mentioned drugs. In view of this it might be interesting that we did not find any increase of tumor formation yet in Germany with intravenous ALG therapy. Some interesting findings based upon animal experiments have been published recently. NELSON was able to show that long lasting ALG application suppresses thymus dependant cellular immune reactions, whereas all thymus dependant antigens cause a normal humoral immune response. That means, that at first the question has to be answered, if the immunological control of tumors is primarily thymus dependent or not.

Summarizing all experimental and clinical studies on immunosuppression and oncogenesis, it can be stated that immunosuppressive treatment favours the formation and growth of malignancies. An exact analysis of the pathomechanism, however, is difficult in humans. The various immunosuppressive procedures have different effects on the immune defense system, while on the other hand a lot of questions are impossible to answer under clinical conditions, so e.g. whether the real tumor producing agents are chemical or viral carcinogens, or if tumor cells have been transplanted together with the grafted organ, or if a latent pre-existent tumor, which was controlled before transplantation, could grow uneffected under immunosuppressive therapy. Anyway, it always will have to be examined if an immunosuppressive procedure has no additional direct oncogenic or leukemogenic effect, or if it is able to influence the tumor as a cytostatic. Table 3 summarizes these effects according to BALNER [16]. As the immunological tumor defense is primarily a cell mediated process [T-cells recognize the tumor cells and killer cells induce the rejection mechanism], in Table 3 only the effects on the cellular immunity are enlisted.

Table 3:
        Effects of immunosuppressive procedures on
                    tumor formation   +]

	standard immunosuppressives		neonatal thymec- tomy	Antilympho- cytic Globuline
	x-rays	Cytostatics		
Effect on cellular immune reaction	+	++	++	+++
Oncogenic resp. leukemogenic effect	++	[+]	-	-
Anti-tumorous and antiproliferative effect	++	++	-	-

+] according to BALNER [16]

Apart from a direct oncogenic effect of some procedures, which possibly potentiates the chemical carcinogenic action, an anti-proliferative effect may exist, which opposes a tumor formation.

In Table 3 only the effects of neonatal thymectomy and of ALG, which is the most powerful suppressive of cell immunity, are enlisted. However, it is difficult to judge the side effects of X-ray-radiation, cytostatics and steroids, because these therapeu-ticals may have tumor potentiating as well as suppressing effects. The whole process is complicated by an indirect oncogenic factor, i.e. the decreased resistance to viral infections due to immuno-suppressive treatment. This effect might be of great importance, because at this moment the diagnosis of carcinogenic viruses in humans is, except in some rare cases, impossible.

Although Azathioprine and steroids were applicated in all cases of human organ transplantation and in some cases the therapy was supplemented by ALS or other immunosuppressives, none of these procedures alone can be held responsible for a particular facilitation of tumor formation with scientific evidence. The animal experiments are of little value in the answer of this question, because - except ALS - there exist no studies with a long time application of Azathioprine and steroids comparable to human transplant recipients. Possibly the continuous antigenic stimulation by the transplanted organ and the bombing of the lymphatic system by immunosuppression and anti-proliferative drugs might be responsible for the formation of reticolo-endo-thelial tumors [GLEICHMANN and GLEICHMANN [42]].

The increased risk of tumor formation by immunosuppressive therapy may therefore till now be explained by the decreased resistance to possibly oncogenic viruses together with a weakened immunological tumor defense, no matter if the tumor itself is caused by viral or chemical carcinogenes.

The most important consequences for clinical organ transplantation should therefore be:

1. To keep the immunosuppressive and antibiotic doses as low as possible,

2. To prefer such immunosuppressives, which have per se no oncogenic effect, and

3. To suppress the humoral, against oncogenic viruses directed antibody formation as little as possible.

Cytostatics - Azathioprine, 6 Mercaptopurine or Methotrexate - don't meet these requirements. ALG, however, has no direct oncogenic effect and despite a powerful effect on the cellular immunity, ALG attenuates the humoral antibody formation to a lesser extent as Azathioprine and other immunosuppressives. Therefore with regards to the tumor risk of an immunosuppressive treatment in organ transplants or autoallergies [diseases with preponderant disorders of cellular immunity], ALG has to be preferred at least as long as the principles of tolerance or enhancement are clinically not available.

References

1. BURNET, F. M. [1959], The Clonal Selection Theory of Acquired Immunity, Cambridge University Press

2. LAW, L. W. [1969], Cancer Res. 29, 1

3. OETTGEN, H. F., OLD, L. J. & BOYSE, E. A. [1971], Med. Clin. North Amer. 55, 761

4. OLD, L. J., BOYSE, E. A., GOERING, G. & OETTGEN, H. F. [1968], Cancer Res. 28, 1288

5. NAGEL, G. A., NAGEL, E., ALBRECHT, R. & BAUDER, E. L. [1975], these Proc.

6. BIRKMAYER, G. P., BALDA, B. R., MILLER, F. & BRAUN-FALCO, O. [1972], Naturwissenschaften 59, 369

7. GÖTZ, H. [1972], Antigenität von Tumorproteinen, Walter de Gruyter, Berlin - New York

8. HELLSTRÖM, I. & HELLSTRÖM, K. E. [1970], Int. J. Cancer 5, 195

9. HELLSTRÖM, I., HELLSTRÖM, K. E., PIERCE, G. E. & YANG, J. P. S. [1968], Nature [London] 220, 1352

10. HELLSTRÖM, I., SJÖGREN, H. O., WARNER, G. & HELLSTRÖM, K. E. [1971], Int. J. Cancer 7, 226

11. ALLISON, A. C., BERMAN, L. D. & LEVEY, R. H. [1967], Nature [London] 215, 185

12. JOHNSON, S. [1968], Brit. J. Cancer 22, 93

13. LAW, L. W. [1965], Cancer Res. 26, 551

14. LAW, L. W. [1965], Nature [London] 205, 672

15. ALLISON, A. C. & LAW, L. W. [1968], Proc. Soc. Exp. Biol. Med. 127, 207

16. BALNER, H. [1970], Europ. J. Clin. Biol. Res. 11, 599

17. BALNER, H. & DERSJANT, H. [1966], J. Nat. Cancer Inst. 36, 513

18. LAW, L. W. [1967], Function of the thymus in tumor induction by viruses, in Perspectives in Virology, vol. 5, chapt. 11, p. 229, N. Y. Academic Press.

19. MILLER, J. F., GRANT, G. A. & ROE, F. J. [1963], Nature [London] 199, 920

20. NISHIZUKA,Y.,KAZUYA,N. & USHI,M.[1965],Nature [London] 205,1236

21. TING,R.C.[1967],Proc.Soc.Exp.Biol.Med. 120,778

22. MARTINEZ,C.[1964],Nature [London] 203,1188

23. CASEY,T.P.[1968],Clin.Exp.Immunol.3, 305

24. JOSEPH,W.L.,MELEWICZ,F.& MORTON,D.L.[1970], Cancer Res. 30,2606

25. HARAN-GHERA,N.[1967],Brit.J.Cancer 21,739

26. HIRSCH,M.S.& MURPHY,F.A.[1968],Lancet 2, 37

27. LAW,L.W.,TING,R.C. & ALLISON,A.C.[1968],Nature [London] 220,611

28. BALNER,H. & DERSJANT,H.[1969],Nature [London] 224,376

29. RABBAT,A.G. & JEEJEEBHOY,H.F.[1970],Transplantation 9,164

30. NELSON,S.[1972],Behring-Inst.Mitt. 51, 201

31. CERRILI,G.J.& TREAT,R.C.[1969],Transplantation 8, 774

32. BALNER,H.[1971],Europ.J.Clin.Biol.Res. 16, 981

33. REIS,H.E.[1972],Z.Krebsforsch.77, 42

34. PENN,I.[1970],Malignant Tumors in Organ-Transplant Recipients, Springer-Verlag, Berlin - Heidelberg -New York

35. PENN,I.& STARZL,T.E.[1972],Transplantation 14, 407

36. STARZL,T.E.[1968],Ann.Surg.168, 416

37. STARZL,T.E.,GROTH,C.G.,BRETTSCHNEIDER,L., SMITH,G.V.,PENN,I. & KASHIWAGI,N.[1969],Antibiot. Chemotherap. 15, 349

38. KUSTER,G.,WOODS,J.E.,ANDERSON,C.F.,WEILAND, L.D. & WILKOWSKE,C.J.[1972],Amer.J.Surgery 123,585

39. MARTIN,D.C.,RUBIN,M. & ROSEN,V.J.[1965],J.Amer. Med.Ass.192, 752

40. WILSON,R.E.,HAGER,E B.,HAMPERS,C.C.,CORSON, J.M.,MERRILL,J.& MURRAY,J.E.[1968],N.Engl.J. Med. 278,479

41. ZUKOSKY,C.E.,KILLEN,D.A.,GIUN,E.,MATTER,B., LUKAS,D.O.& SEIGLER,H.F.[1970],Transplantation 9,71

42. GLEICHMANN,E. & GLEICHMANN,H.[1973],Klin.Wochenschr. 51,260

6.3 Behaviour of GUARINI Reaction in Children with Hemolymphoblastoses and non Tumoral Diseases

L. Benso, N. Nigro, P. Iudicello, R. M. Brunet and R. M. Jacob

In order to study the reaction between human sera and a fraction rich in RNA from a mutant of Saccharomyces Cerevisiae [1-10], children sera obtained from haemolymphoblastoses and other non-neoplastic diseases were examined by the reaction of complement fixation and by electrophoresis, after incubation with or without this fraction. This investigation was conducted parallel with that about the adults, as reported in the preceding paper, which should be consulted for further details.

Methods

Human serum is obtained from fasting subjects, by puncture of elbow vein in older children or jugular vein in younger children. Serum is divided into two samples, one for the reaction of complement fixation and the other for the electrophoretic test. The experiment must be performed not later than few hours after bleeding in order to avoid the spontaneous transformation of $ß_1C$ globulin into $ß_1A$ globulin.

Gel Electrophoresis: The reaction technique used was described in the preceding paper and only main features are described here [10-11].Fresh serum, after incubation with a fraction rich in RNA [$30'/37^{o}C$] was electrophorized [130 Volt-8 mA] on an agar slide [Difco Purified]. As a control, migration of the same serum after incubation with Veronal sodium buffer [pH 7,2] was performed. After electrophoresis, rapid fixation, drying and coloration were carried out. The examination of protidogram thus prepared, may or may not show the disappearance of a band on betaglobulins region [corresponding to $\beta_1 C$ globulin [10]] in incubated sera with the fraction rich in RNA.

Complement fixation: At the same time each serum was examined by the serological method described at the beginning of our work and as the reaction is not well known yet, it will still be called complement fixation, since it is similar in technique with the latter. The technique of reaction was described in detail in several experimental work and only the main features are described here [1 - 4, 7]. The serum was diluted in Veronal sodium buffer 1/10 [pH 7.2]. Complement source is the same serum, titrated before the experiment [7-10] against the haemolytic mixture formed by sheep red cells and rabbit-sheep haemolytic serum.

Cases and Results

282 sera from children aged between two months and 13 years with non-neoplastic diseases of haemolymphoblastoses were tested. Results are shown in Table 1. Table 2 analyses the electrophoretic results of children sera with non-tumoral diseases compared with their age, and children sera with haemolymphoblastoses compared with evolutional stage of their disease. The research showed:

1] In accordance with statistical analysis which shows a significative agreement of 99% [according to x^2 calculation] between two methods, it appears that there are two different methods which test the same phenomenon.

2] The major part of children sera with non-tumoral disease show positive complement fixation and $\beta_1 C$ globulin disappearance by electrophoresis after incubation with a fraction rich in RNA of Saccharomyces Cerevisiae.

Table 1: Behaviour of GUARINI Reaction in Children

	Total	Electrophoresis		Complement Fixation	
		Band disappearance	Band persistence	C.F. positive	C.F. negative
Children	282				
Non-tumoral diseases	210	150 [71,4%]	60 [28,6%]	182 [36,8%]	28[13,4%]
Haemolym-phoblastoses	72	34 [47,2%]	38 [52,8%]	34[47,2%]	38[52,8%]

Table 2: Analysis of Electrophoretic Results

	Cases number	Electrophoresis	
		Band disappear-ance	Band persistence
Non-tumoral cases	210	150 [71,4 %]	60 [28,6 %]
Children under 2 years	34	20 [58,8 %]	14 [41,1 %]
Children above 2 years	176	130 [73,8 %]	46 [26,1 %]
Haemolymphoblastoses	72	34 [47,2 %]	38 [52,8 %]
Remission [1]	38	26 [68,42%]	12 [31,57 %]
Absence of remission	34	8 [23,52%]	26 [76,47%]

[1] Remissive Haemolymphoblastoses characterized by: absence of clinic and radiological findings, normalization of sedimentation rate, normal blood formula, bone marrow blasts under 5%.

- --------

3] The major part of children sera with haemolymphoblastosis show negative complement fixation and $\beta_1 C$ globulin persistence by the same experiment.

4] These differences may appear less significant for children than for adults, however, if results are compared with age, it appears that with children over two years old, disappearance percentage of band is usually comparable with that of adults, but in children under two years old the disappearance frequency of the band is lower.

5] Children with haemolymphoblastoses [all over two years] were similar to non-neoplastic patients during the period of remission, but children in acute phase of disease or children with incomplete clinical remission displayed a very considerable persistence of the band.

Discussion

The possible interpretations of the mechanism of the phenomenon is not clear. In short, results may suggest that RNA of a Sacharomyces Cerevisiae mutant causes the transformation of β_1C globulin fraction into β_1A [which have a different electrophoretic migration], and it occurs in all healthy subjects or in children over two years old with non-neoplastic disease. This transformation is much less frequent in sera of children younger than two years and does not happen in the majority of sera of children with haemolymphoblastoses.

Summary: By agar electrophoretic method the authors show disappearance of a band corresponding to beta globulins in the protidogram of children with non-tumoral disease, after incubation with RNA of Saccharomyces Cerevisiae. On the other hand the beta globulin band persists in sera of children with haemolymphoblastoses.

References

1. SERRA, A., GUARINI, G., LOVISETTO, P., CASTELLO, D. & BALZOLA, F. [1958], Nature [London] 181, 622

2. BARBU, E. & DANDEU, C.R. [1963], C.R. Acad. Sci. Paris 256,. 2948

3. SERRA, A., GUARINI, G., GUIDETTI, E., MAISIN, J. & DECKERS, Ch. [1965], Nature [London] 206, 1264

4. SERRA, A., GUARINI, G., GUIDETTI, E., MAISIN, J. & DECKERS, Ch. [1965], Nature [London] 206, 1266

5. MAISIN, J., GUARINI, G., LOVISETTO, P., SERRA, A. & GUIDETTI, E. [1967], Bull. Acad. Roy Med. Belgique 7, 289

6. LOVISETTO, P., MOLFESE, G., BOGGIATO, A., BIARESE, V. & GUARINI, G. [1968], La Presse Med. 76, 1327

7. NIGRO, N., GUARINI, G., BENSO, L., MADON, E., IUDICELLO, P. & JACOB, R.M. [1971], La Presse Med. 79, 227

8. LOVISETTO, P., MOLFESE, G., BOGGIATO, A., BIARESE, V., GUARINI, G. & VISCONTI, A. [1969], La Presse Med. 77, 1383

9. BENSO, L., GUARINI, G., NIGRO, N., IUDICELLO, P., JACOB, R.M., FERRARI, G. & BARONCELLI, P. [1971], XII Congr. Int. Pediatria, Vienna, p. 59

10. DECKERS, Ch. & GUARINI, G. [1971], Prot. Biol. Fluids Proc. 18th Colloq., Pergamon Press, Oxford - New York

11. MAISIN, J., COUVREUR, P., OCHRYMOWICZ, I.P. & Van DYSE, E. [1972], Europ. J. Cancer 8, 217